The Future of Medicare?
Health Innovation in 21st Century Australia

Edited with Introduction by
JEREMY SAMMUT

David Gadiel Jessica Borbasi Peta Seaton Gerald Thomas

Special Publication 13

THE CENTRE FOR
INDEPENDENT
STUDIES

2018

Connor Court Publishing

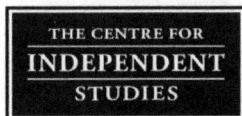

Published June 2018
by The Centre for Independent Studies Limited and Connor Court Publishing Pty Ltd

The Centre for Independent Studies Limited
Level 1, 131 Macquarie Street, Sydney NSW 2000
Email: cis@cis.org.au
Website: www.cis.org.au

Connor Court Publishing Pty Ltd,
Po Box 7257, Redland Bay, 4165
Email: sales@connorcourt.com
Website: www.connorcourtpublishing.com.au

ISBN 9781925826043

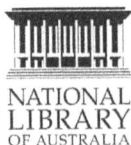

Table of Contents

CHAPTER 3:
Health Innovation Communities

CHAPTER 4:
Consumer-Directed Aged Care

CHAPTER 6:

CHAPTER 7:

List of Figures

The Future of Medicare?

Health Innovation in 21st Century Australia

The Centre for Independent Studies acknowledges
the support of the Thyne Reid Foundation for the
Health Innovations Program

thynereid
FOUNDATION

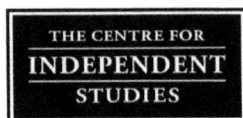

THE CENTRE FOR
INDEPENDENT
STUDIES

Chapter 1

Introduction

Jeremy Sammut

Quo Vadis Medicare?

Medicare—Australia's $74 billion-plus taxpayer-funded, universal healthcare scheme—has remained largely unchanged since its inception in 1984. If this continues, Medicare will continue to support a nineteenth-century craft style model of healthcare, underwritten by a twentieth-century command-and-control style funding system. Medicare will primarily continue to pay doctors for delivering a defined medical service in the form of a one-off episode of mainly GP or other specialist and hospital care on a fee-for-service basis. The problem with this traditional model of medical and hospital care is that it was more suited to earlier times when the bulk of the Australian community's health needs consisted of short-term treatment for acute illness. It is less suited to dealing with the number one health challenge of the twenty-first century: the effective treatment and management of the rising burden of chronic disease in an ageing Australia.

This book is a collection of chapters dealing with different aspects of the most 'wicked' policy and political challenge the country faces: the future of Medicare. Its first objective is to get the reader to basecamp on the Everest of Australian health reform. The problems with the current structure of Medicare, outlined here, suggest we should chart a new direction in health, and make changes to a system that is widely considered the jewel in the crown of Australian social policy—along with being the third-rail of Australian politics, given the electorates' well-demonstrated conservatism regarding Medicare.

If the status quo prevails, and we do not overcome the formidable political obstacles to doing things differently in health, Medicare will not only become increasingly unaffordable. Medicare will also be unable to meet the health needs of Australians in the most responsive and patient-centred way, and will be unable to adapt and innovate to meet the most pressing challenges threatening the quality and sustainability of Australian healthcare. This book therefore presents the case for modernising the way Medicare funds and delivers health services to the Australian community, and proposes a series of politically-feasible reform options and strategies to implement innovative health policy and healthcare solutions for the problems that Medicare faces in coming decades.

The major problem, in practice, with the way Medicare functions today , is that under the current set of Medicare payments and services, too much is spent on some kinds of often very expensive healthcare, and not enough on different kinds of services that could both contain health expenditure and improve health outcomes for patients. As explained in Chapter 2, we spend more than we should on costly hospital-based care for chronic disease patients, and not enough on non-hospital primary care that could keep people well and avoid hospital admissions. This is attributed to the 'gaps' prevalent in the doctor-and-hospital-centric Medicare system for chronic disease care—defined as a lack of access to a full range of community-based, multidisciplinary, medical, nursing, and allied healthcare.

These structural problems—which raise the cost and lower the quality of Australian healthcare—are well-recognised in the health policy debate. Insights into the limitations of Medicare have been stated and re-stated in countless reports, reviews and inquiries into health policy and reform. The latest reiteration of these findings can be found in the December 2015 report of Primary Health Care Advisory Group commissioned by the federal government, which was indicatively titled *Better Outcomes for People with Chronic and Complex Health Conditions.*[1] The health policy debate also features lots of theoretical talk about what may sound like a relatively easy fix. Many health experts and stakeholders agree the sustainability of Medicare can be improved by redesigning and integrating health services across the sector to deliver different types of care, at different times, in different places; to deliver lower-cost primary care services that could help the chronically-ill avoid requiring high-cost hospital services.*

However, the reality is that all the talk of redesigning the system to better manage chronic disease and minimise use of hospitals is easier said than done, because of the rigid, inflexible, and provider-centric nature of Medicare's traditional service and payment systems. Rather than a comprehensive health insurance system, in reality, Medicare primarily functions as a series of provider-captured payments for separate sets of community-based primary care and hospital-based care, which principally and perpetually reward GPs and other specialists, corporate medical clinics, and public hospitals for delivering the same old traditional model of one-off services and unintegrated care in the same old way. This means Medicare is not a health 'system' per se, because that term implies a spectrum of integrated, patient-centred services that deliver the best and most cost-effective health outcomes.

This also means that under the current Medicare structure, it is impossible to reallocate existing Medicare funding—even funding that is used wastefully or sub-optimally—in order to implement innovative models of integrated healthcare. Because there is no existing Medical Benefit Scheme (MBS) benefit, or case-mix 'activity-based' payment, or other existing stream of program funding associated with these new models, those who might develop those alternative models about which there is so much theoretical discussion are defeated by the 'system'. Innovators cannot utilise any of the tens-of-billions of dollars that are locked up in the existing service and payment framework. And perversely, from the perspective of governments and policymakers, new ideas that could improve outcomes and save money loom as additive —potential extra cost— and are therefore not implemented.

---

* For but one example, see the 'Innovation in Healthcare Roundtable' hosted by The Australian Financial Review in November 2016: the consensus was that "our health system needs to be re-engineered to better meet the needs of the future", and that "real innovation will come from a more integrated, more coordinated approach to health service delivery across the sector", which will "provide prevention and treatment at the optimum time for patients and the community." http://www.afr.com/news/special-reports/future-of-healthcare/health-system-strong-in-some-areas-but-lacking-policy-innovation-20161106-gsj1co

Bending the cost curve down...and beyond

The structural problems in Medicare—and the structural barriers to healthcare innovation—portend an ominous future of less national wellness and prosperity in coming decades. It suggests health expenditure will continue to escalate on the high-cost hospital treatment for increasing numbers of chronic patients with complex conditions who could potentially be better and more efficiently cared for outside hospital.

The scale of these problems is indicated by the fact that an estimated 10% of hospital admissions each year are classified as 'potentially preventable' had patients received prior, effective primary care services. This estimate of hundreds-of-thousands of avoidable admissions costing Medicare hundreds-of-millions of dollars per annum is even more significant, given that an estimated 5–10% of patients are heavy users of health services, and account for 50% of healthcare costs across the system.[2] Many of these patients are those chronic disease sufferers with complex medical conditions who are the so-called 'frequent flyers' requiring repeated and lengthy stays in hospitals. Large savings on overall health expenditure could thus be achieved by more efficient and effective management of these patients across the whole value chain in health—including primary care, pharmaceuticals and hospital services. Hence, conservative estimates suggest that the well-known structural inefficiencies in Australian healthcare currently cost the nation more than $17.7 billion a year—11% of the total national health spend—across the $161.6 billion Australian (public and private[†]) health system.[3]

Focusing on the financial implications of Medicare is the standard way in which health policy challenges are discussed. Emphasising the need to bend the forecast health cost curve downwards to limit the impact on the public finances has been the approach adopted by successive federal governments via the Intergenerational Reports (IGR) periodically prepared by the Federal

---

† Taxpayers bear the cost of inefficiencies in health. But so do private health fund members through the increased cost of insurance premiums. In parallel fashion to the problems in Medicare, health funds have very limited ability to control their costs due to the highly-regimented character of the private health insurance sector in Australia as discussed in Chapters 2 and 3.

Treasury, which have modelled the impact of current health (and other) policy settings on the federal budget over the next 40 years.

The fourth Intergenerational Report was released by the Abbott government in March 2015 and delivered the same message as the previous three. IGR4 outlined how the status quo in health, combined with the impact on health costs of the unprecedented ageing of the population, will make Medicare fiscally unsustainable, as the cost of the scheme will not be able to be funded out of existing sources of revenue without imposing significant tax hikes on future generations. Yet the IGRs have generated little momentum for policy change. The theme of long-term unaffordability—crucial though it is to the nation's finances—simply has not gained traction in the public mind as a stimulus and justification for significant changes to Medicare.

The political implications for health reform are crucial. Health funding remains the single largest budgetary challenge facing Australian governments, and will in the long-run exhaust government's ability to tax and spend on health. But the theme of unsustainable cost to government budgets is clearly insufficient – and probably counter-productive – in terms of framing and promoting health reform purely in economic terms. (Particularly when, in the contemporary political lexicon, the term 'reform' has become a dirty word synonymous with 'cuts' and the creation of 'losers'.) Given the limitations of the current Medicare system, the questions pertaining to health reform can more persuasively be framed through the prism of innovation—in terms of focusing on the benefits for consumers, taxpayers, and the community of doing things differently in health, such as addressing the problems with traditional service and payment models that impede the development of new and better ways of delivering healthcare. This is the approach—the new paradigm for advocating health reform —applied in the chapters in this book, which were first published as research reports by The Centre for Independent Studies' Health Innovations Program.

Herein also lies the way to make the case for change in terms of the potential *social* benefits of health reform. Medicare currently works well for people with less complex health needs: if you have a simple problem, Medicare offers a straightforward, one-off solution; but if people have complex problems, they confront a complex system. For chronic disease patients, the health system is fragmented and difficult to navigate; patients from lower socio-economic groups may also miss out on complete necessary care due both to service gaps—the fact that Medicare does not in many cases cover the full cost of the full cycle of treatment—and due to poor health literacy and self-management skills. Higher health expenditure and sub-optimal wellbeing for the poorest and sickest patients results from there being no single funder, no single provider, being accountable for the entire healthcare of the whole person and for the overall cost and health outcomes, regardless of where that care is delivered.

The 'Solution': Capitation & Integration

Dealing with these structural challenges is not simply a matter of governments and health departments adding new Medicare-funded 'care coordination' services, as is routinely suggested. As Chapter 2 shows, there is scant evidence this kind of 'top down' (additive and bureaucratically-run) approach to so-called innovative healthcare is effective and actually prevents hospital admissions. Instead, the fundamental defect that needs to be addressed are the incentives and associated institutional impediments that currently prevail across the Medicare system and prevent the delivery of integrated care. Medicare is an input driven system that rewards providers on the basis of activity—for the volume of discrete health interventions delivered, regardless of the results attained. Providers are not financially or otherwise accountable for the overall health outcomes achieved, nor are they responsible for managing the healthcare of patients across the spectrum of services in a cost-effective manner to achieve improvements in health status and wellbeing. In practice, the fragmented fee-for-service funding for GP, other medical, and hospital services means there is little financial incentive across the system to stop a patient coming to hospital.

Once again, identifying the problem suggests the solution: an alternative funding model, known as capitated payments that might 'pool' existing federal and state health and hospital funding,‡ and allocate funding to a specified healthcare provider on a per person basis. Capitated funding would give providers the flexibility and (currently lacking) incentive to innovate and reallocate resources more efficiently and effectively to reduce costs and improve outcomes. Capitated funding would make providers financially responsible for funding the care of patients across the full service spectrum. It would therefore allow and encourage providers to develop innovative and cost-effective integrated models of care—to basically front-load spending that otherwise would fund hospital care, to develop new services to better manage chronic disease more effectively outside hospital, and ensure patients receive the most appropriate treatment in the lowest cost setting.

But achieving this kind of systemic 'solution' is no simple matter, as the political obstacles to meaningful health reform are formidable. Because Medicare guarantees the income and supports the business model of existing providers, the politics of health are replete with entrenched vested interests determined to protect the status quo. (Hence Medicare is better described as a 'political economy' rather than a health system.) The size of the impediments to reform can be measured by the response to even relatively minor changes to Medicare. The Abbott government's ill-fated $7 mandatory GP co-payment proposal of 2014—which was designed to address the inherent moral hazard and over-use of health services that occurs in a 'free' health system (see below)—was defeated due to community opposition led and orchestrated by the organised medical profession. The Australian Medical Association (AMA) is also vehemently opposed to any move towards capitated funding—which is routinely and emotively branded as a step towards 'US-style Managed Care' or the 'Americanisation' of the health system. Medicare's status as an untouchable 'sacred cow' has been reinforced by the Labor Party's successful 'Mediscare' during the 2016 federal election—the false claim the

---

‡ For those unfamiliar with the full jurisdictional complexity of Australia's complex division of health responsibilities between federal and state government's under Australia's federation: medical services provided outside hospitals are the principal responsibility of the federal government and receive separate federal funding on a fee-for-service, open-ended basis. Federal money also partially funds the operation of public hospitals—on condition that all Australians are entitled to receive 'free' public hospital care at point of access. State and territory governments are responsible for hospital governance and administration.

Coalition was intent on privatising Medicare—which proved an important factor contributing to the loss of support for the Turnbull government.[4]

Politically-Feasible Reform

The chances of achieving meaningful health reform may therefore appear slim – especially the likelihood of achieving 'big bang' reforms. This includes the 'Medicare Select' proposal favoured by many stakeholders in the private health insurance industry, which would convert Medicare into a 'voucher system' allowing all Australians to purchase private health plans. The odds against implementing such root-and-branch transformation are great, despite the merits and potential benefits of the Medicare Select model of system-wide change to the way taxpayer funding is used to purchase the most appropriate and cost-effective healthcare for Australians (see Chapter 2).[5]

Moreover, because workable ways and detailed strategy to overcome the political obstacles are rarely, if ever, set out even by supporters of change, much of the health policy and health reform debate in this country is tantamount to simply being besotted with endlessly talking about the problems in the health system. This book is different: it sets out a politically-feasible way to initiate health reform, implement health service payment and service integration, and catalyse healthcare innovation.

Chapter 3 outlines a plan to establish 'Health Innovation Communities' in Australia. Health Innovation Communities (HICs) are based on the concept of free trade zones, which have been used throughout history to relax existing cultural norms and laws, and remove disincentives to trade and commerce and the development of new modes of doing business. What I and my co-authors, Peta Seaton and Gerald Thomas, have proposed is that within designated geographic regions declared to be HICs, consumers and providers would be free to choose to opt-in to a capitated payment model and integrated service system.

Within HIC-declared areas, healthcare providers could apply for exemptions from existing Medicare (and private health insurance legislation) and be allowed to create and use alternative payment and service delivery models that are currently banned. Exempt providers — including companies, start-up entrepreneurs, charities, private health funds, and federal and state government health agencies — could then recruit individuals who wish to voluntarily opt-in to receive integrated care – supported by a funding model that pooled federal and state funding (and private health funding where appropriate). Capitated funding would give providers the (much needed) flexibility and incentive to innovate and integrate; reallocating resources more efficiently to cost-effectively manage patient care across the full service spectrum to improve health outcomes. This would also include discovering better ways to manage utilisation and the current latently inefficient over-use of hospital services — and thereby address Australia's very high rates of hospital use compared to the OECD, by substituting high-cost hospital-based procedures, images, and tests with lower-cost community clinics for specialist treatment.

What makes HICs politically viable is that a system of "Silicon Valley" hubs for healthcare research, development and innovation would leave the current Medicare (and private health insurance) entitlements and payment and service arrangements intact for the vast majority of health consumers and providers. This would move the debate beyond the toxic, innovation-killing politics of health – and minimise the impact of 'Mediscare' tactics —— as exemptions from the existing rules would be permitted only within dedicated regions and apply only to those consumers and providers within HICs who choose to opt-in to the new arrangements. This would respect the public support for Medicare for those who want to choose Medicare, while respecting the choice of those who might want to choose an alternative to the existing (compulsory) Medicare framework.

It might be argued that similar change is already occurring in the health sector. As Chapter 3 notes, the federal government's 'Health Care Home' program has taken preliminary steps towards creating a capitation funding mechanism for chronic care. However, a mere $120 million has been committed to three-year Health Care Home trial — a mere drop in the health funding bucket. Based on the size of this so-called 'investment' in *trialling* innovative models of care, no existing provider is likely to risk (or bother) disrupting their established Medicare-funded business model. A national health innovation strategy focused on HICs, by contrast, would send a clear signal that Australian governments are serious about innovation, by adding much greater scale to existing initiatives to integrate care, and by giving many more innovators the opportunity to enter the market and discover new and better ways of delivering services.

The key to the concept is that HICs will create an environment, an eco-system, in which novel healthcare products and solutions can emerge from the bottom up. Within HICs, a plurality of innovators will have the opportunity to develop and refine different models at the coal-face of patient care to achieve the best financial and health outcomes. This discovery and knowledge-creation process would allow competing models to be simultaneously tested against each other — in a real world, competitive and contestable commercial setting — once existing structural shackles are released. The opportunities that HICs open up for innovation will demonstrate the benefits of doing things differently in health. Once functioning models were established, and were proven to use scarce health resources more efficiently, effectively, and sustainably, they could provide workable blueprints for change that could be rolled out system-wide. If these models work well and achieve better outcomes in a HIC, why not in the rest of the country?

A Parable for Medicare

Even HICs might seem a step too far away from the status quo to be genuinely feasible at a time when both sides of politics are more interested in offering 'guarantees' that no significant changes will be made to Medicare.[§] However, to place the HIC proposal (and what may actually be possible) in context, innovation — or the lack thereof — in the health sector should be compared against reforms in comparable social service sectors that face similar cost, policy, and service delivery challenges.

---

§ To this effect, the Turnbull Government created the "Medicare Guarantee Fund" in the 2017 Budget to fund the MBS and PBS in perpetuity, with the political aim of neutralising Labor's 'Mediscare'.

The federal government's recently implemented 'Consumer-Directed Care' (CDC) aged care reforms are of great significance as they offer an important opportunity to demonstrate the benefits of reform to often sceptical and change-averse members of the public. Under the new CDC system, each ageing Australian requiring home-based aged care and support services can now access an individualised funding budget (according to their assessed level of need) to purchase the type, mix and provider of services they want, based on personal choice. CDC 'packages' replaced the long-established system of block funding of 'Approved Providers' via competitive tender. Similar to the situation under the current rigid structure of Medicare—whereby consumers essentially have to take what providers are specifically funded to deliver —the now-defunct, highly-regimented aged care funding system limited the consumer's choice to the kind of one-size-fits-all service model providers chose to offer. This invariably took the form of a standardised set of services involving centralised rostering of head office managers of care workers, who rotate in and out of homes and perform set tasks in a set time frame.

The key objective of the CDC reforms is to increase the flexibility and responsiveness of the system to meet the personal needs and diverse expectations of increasingly demanding consumers. Empowering consumers of aged care services with the freedom to choose creates incentive for providers to tailor their range of services to suit the recipient's individual needs, in order to win the custom of those who are free to take their business elsewhere. The introduction of choice and competition is also designed to spur providers to discover operational efficiencies and other innovations that can increase the amount, and mix, of frontline services delivered. Chapter 4 outlines that this process of disruption is being driven by the CDC reforms new and technologically innovative 'Uber'-style online platforms – that have far less costly head office overheads compared to traditional providers that waste between a third to half of all funding on administrative fees - to enter the market and deliver more than double the amount of personalised care out of the same level of funding than traditional providers.

Herein lies a parable for Medicare: reforms that move away from traditional provider-centric, highly regulated and inflexible models of care can generate better value, better quality, and better outcomes for both consumers and for governments. HICs, which would inject the dynamic principles of choice and competition into the health sector, have the potential to achieve similar results for chronic disease care that the CDC reforms can for aged care. The further lesson to draw from the CDC reforms is the way bi-partisan political support was generated for change. Following extensive community consultation, lobbying and support by aged advocacy groups, and persistent expressions of dissatisfaction with the status quo from consumers and their families, policymakers chose to put the needs of older Australians (and taxpayers) ahead of the vested interests of established providers. A grass-roots campaign for HICs could tap into similar sentiments and mobilise the potential support and demand for change among chronic disease sufferers and patient advocacy groups, who might want to choose an alternative to Medicare's rigidities and limitations that could deliver more and better healthcare.

As stated above, we should be wary of calls for another health inquiry and report process. Yet a broad-based, independent review of the Australian health system conducted by the Productivity Commission (see Chapter 2) could serve a constructive purpose with certain provisos, given the important role the Commission's work has played in stimulating consumer-based reform in the disability and aged care services sectors. However, to promote a similar outcome with regards to health policy, a Productivity Commission inquiry will need to do more than simply describe the problems in the system; any recommendations forthcoming from the inquiry will also have to extend far beyond proposing 'solutions' limited to piecemeal trials of integrated payment and care programs.[6] Nonetheless, a Productivity Commission inquiry remains the right forum in which to foster greater awareness among policymakers and the general public of the changing needs of consumers in the new age of chronic disease, and to promote the potential benefits of innovation within the health sector to meet the communities evolving and more complex healthcare needs. But—to reiterate—another health inquiry will only serve a useful purpose if the policy recommendations developed by the Commission are practical, achievable and meaningful—which is the criteria the HIC proposal is purpose-built to fit.

Chapter 5 extends the discussion of why and how things need to be done differently in health: Dr Jessica Borbasi provides a specific example of how the rigidities of the health system compromise quality care, and how a more flexible approach would also improve cost-effectiveness of health services with regards the crucial subject of palliative care.

Palliative care—properly defined—is a form of coordinated, patient-centred, 'team care' that is proven to not only alleviate pain, but to improve the quality of life of patients suffering incurable chronic illness in the later and last stages of life. As Borbasi shows, the need for greater access to palliative care services in Australia is being generated by the success of the 'treat and cure' health system in resolving short-term illness, prolonging life, and contributing significantly to the rapid ageing of the population. However, as Borbasi also shows, this reactive model of healthcare is not fit for purpose to deal with the consequences of the modern medical revolution —the new realities of modern death that will see the majority of Australians die at very old ages from multiple, chronic 'diseases of ageing'. As a result, dying patients in Australia do not receive the kind of care they need and want, but the kind of care the system is presently set up to deliver: disjointed, inflexible and non-holistic care, often involving frequent hospital admissions and intensive 'curative' interventions.

This can lead to the kind of over-medicalised—and often distressing and painful—death that is feared by many in the community, but which a wealth of evidence shows that good palliative care can prevent. To ensure that the dual ethical and economic challenges of increasing access to palliative care are addressed, Borbasi argues that an 'investment approach' needs to be adopted by the government to calculate the real cost of unintegrated 'end of life' care across the health system and whole of government, and use this information to drive service and funding redesigns that support evidence-based palliative services. Borbasi's recommendations suggest that policymakers should look towards more market-based and consumer-centred solutions, potentially through a commissioning approach to palliative care services.

Controlling the Real Cost of Health

Chapters 2, 3, 4, and 5 examine innovation on the *supply-side* of Medicare: how providers of health services can be encouraged and enabled to deliver more and better quality and value healthcare to Australians by using available resources more efficiently and effectively for the benefit of both consumers and governments' bottom line. Chapters 6, 7 and 8 discuss innovation on the *demand-side* of Medicare: how individuals can be encouraged to be more cost-conscious users of health services by assuming greater personal financial responsibility for healthcare financing.

Demand-side health reform challenges the core principle of Medicare: that universal access to healthcare should be paid for by taxes and be consumed for 'free'. Like all traditional health systems in countries like Australia that rely heavily on third-party private or public insurance to pay for the bulk of health services, Medicare is plagued by 'moral hazard' — the problem of over-use of insured health services for doubtful health gain. Due to the absence of price signals — direct charges to patients at point of consumption — demand for Medicare-funded health services will inevitably grow faster than supply, leading to a demand-cost-and-tax-spiral that is the root cause of the ever-escalating cost of health.

In terms of addressing these demand-side challenges, the abandonment of the Abbott government's Medicare co-payment teaches important lessons about voters' attitudes towards Medicare, and the political challenges of health reform. The public health lobby presented the rejection of the co-payment as a symbol of the popular commitment to the 'fairness' of Medicare and the principle of universal access to 'free' healthcare funded by taxes. More telling, however, was the Labor Party's description of the co-payment as a 'GP Tax'. The co-payment — which would have introduced a very modest element of means-tested, compulsory and direct cost-sharing into the Medicare system to control the use and limit the cost of GP and other medical services—proved an easy political kill because Medicare's popularity is actually underwritten by an understandable 'hip-pocket' sentiment. Consuming 'free' healthcare is one the most obvious ways that many people feel they get recompense for paying taxes to government. Hence the level of bulk billing—the percentage of GP visits that incur no additional fee charged to patients (currently 85%[7]) — has from some become a political touchstone and yardstick of whether Medicare is considered to be operating effectively.

The irony of this entitlement mentality is that it is based on a fiscal fiction that tricks people into believing they are slugged only a small percentage of their incomes to pay for Medicare: most taxpayers do not actually realise how much tax they are truly paying to fund the system. The myth is that the 1.5% Medicare Levy[¶] on personal taxable income—which is paid by all income earners, with exemptions for aged pensioners and the low-incomed— funds Medicare. In reality, the revenue raised by the Medicare Levy covers a mere fraction of the cost of health. In 2014-15, the levy raised $10.75 billion and covered just 14.3% of the $74.7 billion cost to Australian governments of the three main Medicare entitlements programs: the Medical Benefits Scheme (MBS), the Pharmaceuticals Benefits Scheme (PBS), and free treatment in public hospitals. To raise the full amount of income tax that covered the full cost of Medicare (which actually accounted for 44% of total income tax), the 'real' Medicare Levy rate would have been 10.4%. Many taxpayers were therefore effectively paying a '10% levy' on their incomes to pay for Medicare.[8]

Such are the contradictions and unrealistic community expectations that lie behind popular support for Medicare. On the one hand, the more 'free' health care that is consumed, the higher taxes need to rise to fund the scheme; the higher the taxes paid, the more 'free' health care is demanded. On the other hand, if governments were more transparent about the real cost of Medicare to taxpayers, the illusions surrounding 'free' healthcare

¶ Note: since July 2014 the Medicare and NDIS Levy has been set at 2%, with the additional 0.5% levied to fund the roll out of the National Disability Insurance Scheme.

might dissipate. Voters might question what they are getting for what they are paying, and might look more favourably on alternatives to the status quo. Drawing attention to the demand-cost-and-tax spiral in health, and making explicit the link between lower tax and controlling health spending, could even encourage voters to see the sense in the use of price signals and co-payments to control health costs and improve Medicare's sustainability.

In Chapter 6, David Gadiel examines how governments have sought to manage the policy and political challenges posed by the undeliverable promise of 'free and universal' access to healthcare. He traces the history of faltering government efforts that have pursued oscillating, paradoxical and inconsistent strategies designed, in turn, to encourage bulk billing, attempt to introduce co-payments to restrict growth in Medicare expenditure, and control the setting of doctor's fees to limit out-of-pocket charges to patients. Gadiel argues that the multiple irrationalities besetting this health policy area could be resolved by a reformed and simplified Medicare system, which made it clear that the government was not in the business of regulating doctor's fees. By abolishing the *Medicare Schedule Fee*, and thereby clarifying that Medicare payments for medical services are purely a 'benefit', the setting of doctor's fees and the charging of GP co-payments and 'gap' payments by specialists would clearly become the business of doctors and patients. Doctors would be free to opt to accept the 'benefit' (aka 'bulk bill') as full payment for their services, or could choose to charge a co-payment, which would be determined and negotiated in a competitive market for medical services.

Chapter 7 extends the focus on the demand-side of Medicare in the health policy area that has been most intractably plagued by the insoluble dilemma of trying to increase 'free' access to healthcare while containing the cost of a 'free' system: state government-owned and operated public hospitals.

Gadiel and I argue that supply-side policies alone— measures that seek to improve the efficiency of health services and value achieved for health spending, such as the national activity-based hospital funding system—will be unable to limit unaffordable growth in the cost of Australia's fundamentally unsustainable 'free' public hospital systems in coming decades. The size of the 'hospital funding gap' is indicated by state government's continued unrealistic calls for the federal government to increase the GST from 10% to 15% to fund the long term cost of hospitals – a 50% tax hike that would be the largest single peacetime taxation increase in history. We argue that rather than praying for a non-existing magic funding pudding to save state budgets from the crippling cost of Medicare, revision of the federation is needed to enable state governments to undertake the demand-side policies essential for sustainable hospital services. By taking back their income tax powers to fund their own health services, state governments would reclaim full control over both funding and policy responsibility, be released from their obligations under Medicare, and no longer be forced to provide 'free' public hospital services as a condition for receiving federal health funding.

We also argue that because the political responsibility for state income taxes (that would rise and fall as necessary to meet the cost of public hospitals) would lie with state governments, states would hereby be encouraged—in order to limit taxes, and subject to the will of their electorates—to implement the rational cost-sharing policies currently not able to be implemented under the rigid Medicare framework. Exposing state taxpayers to the true cost of 'free' hospital would also encourage voters—in return for lower taxes—to be open to the 'hard conversation' about the future of public hospitals and accept the introduction of a compulsory co-payment to better manage demand for, and cost of, hospital treatment.

We also argue that such a 'courageous' assault on the fundamentals of Medicare is electorally viable by introducing compulsory hospital co-payments in a novel 'revenue neutral' fashion. Ordinary citizens can be convinced to take greater personal responsibility for helping curb health costs (and without price signals deterring necessary use of hospitals) by the government automatically paying all households in that state, quarterly compensation equivalent to the actuarial cost of a typical household's expected co-payment charges—regardless of whether they actually used a public hospital service. The cost of the compensation would be recouped by revenue generated by the co-payment, and by savings generated by reducing unnecessary use of hospital services. The combined impact of state income taxes and hospital co-payments would encourage states and citizens to pursue lower-cost, non-hospital treatment options, and thereby create a political environment amenable to healthcare innovation and facilitating the creation of HICs.

This chapter also recognises that achieving universal agreement among the states on reform of the federation would be difficult. Ideally, states could individually and voluntarily reclaim their income tax powers and authority over health policy, in conjunction with a tax swap with the federal government. This path—the federal government striking differential rates of income taxes across states—is unconstitutional, as sections 99 and 51(ii) of the Australian Constitution prohibit unequal treatment of states by the Commonwealth with respect to taxation. However, optional reform of the federation on a state-by-state basis is still possible under the indirect but constitutionally valid plan outlined in the chapter. This would convert federal health funding into indexed general purpose payments for public hospital services, the value of which would be identified with the equivalent percentage of federal income collected in the state—thereby creating a 'public hospital levy' that states would be free to adjust by imposing their own income tax surcharge or rebate.

Opt-Out Health Savings Accounts

Average per-person total federal, state and territory government spending on health currently sits at close to $4600 per annum. This considerable sum—the 'hidden cost' of Medicare—presents an opportunity to implement another innovative, choice-based potential solution to the nation's health policy and political challenges. Chapter 8 outlines another way to encourage individuals to assume greater personal responsibility for health – and to directly benefit from a superior alternative to Medicare.

Gadiel and I argue that individuals should be allowed to opt-out of Medicare. This would involve converting the funding that would otherwise fund Medicare into a yearly, indexed 'voucher' for deposit in a superannuation-style, tax-advantaged health savings account. The money in these accounts would be able to be withdrawn to pay for an approved list of lower-cost health services. Health Savings Accounts would also pay for private health insurance premiums to cover chronic and catastrophic conditions, and thereby meet the high-cost of hospital admissions and major illness, as well as pay for co-payments and deductibles applying to insured services.

Medicare opt-outs represent a politically viable pathway to health reform for the same reason as HICs: those who wanted to stay with Medicare would be free to do so and their entitlements would be unaltered. But those who want an alternative would be free to choose. However, the real political key to Medicare opt-out health savings accounts is that it offers individuals something far better than getting their taxes back through Medicare.

The key to health savings accounts is the common sense principle that because people will be spending their own money to purchase more of their own healthcare, they will always spend that money more wisely than a government or private insurance benefit, since they stand to directly and personally benefit financially from using their own health dollars in a cost-conscious fashion. Singapore spends around half the proportion of national income on health (4.9% of GDP in 2014) than Australia (10% of GDP in 2014-15) while achieving the same or better health outcomes, due to its national system of health savings accounts. The consequent use of prices, cost-sharing and direct patient charges across the whole healthcare spectrum, funded either out of health savings accounts or as out-of-pocket charges, is an example of how personal financial responsibility for health expenditures contains health costs and increases health system affordability by encouraging citizens to make judicious choices about use of health services.

Under the opt-out health savings account system outlined in Chapter 7, the financial incentives to consume health services wisely and affordably would be enhanced by linking personal health savings accounts to individuals' superannuation accounts in retirement (as occurs in Singapore). This would enable the 'health savings' generated by responsible consumption of healthcare to be used to pay for both old age health costs and to increase retirement incomes. The benefits of withdrawing from Medicare and assuming personal responsibility for self-funding their own health care would not simply only flow to government budgets. Health savings accounts would undoubtedly enhance the sustainability of Australian healthcare by creating off-budget sources of health funding. Health savings accounts would also be the most effective way to address the healthcare use and cost spiral that endangers health system sustainability. However, the real winners from this innovative model of health reform would be the individuals who opt out of Medicare and reap the rewards—higher health savings account balances and ultimately higher retirement incomes—of choosing a lower-cost and financially rewarding way to pay for better health care.

Endnotes

1   http://www.health.gov.au/internet/main/publishing.nsf/Content/76B2BDC12AE54540CA257F72001102B9/$File/Primary-Health-Care-Advisory-Group_Final-Report.pdf

2   Council of Australian Governments. Heads of Agreement between the Commonwealth and the States on Public Hospital Funding. 1 Apr 2016. http://www.coag.gov.au/sites/default/files/communique/Heads%20of%20Agreement%20between%20the%20Commonwealth%20and%20the%20States%20on%20Public%20Hospital%20Funding%20-%201%20April%202016.pdf

3   See Chapter 3.

4   Jeremy Sammut, 'Health – Opt-Out of Medicare and Opt-In for Personal Health Savings Accounts' in James Allan (ed.), Making Australia Right, (Brisbane: Connor Court, 2017).

5   http://www.theaustralian.com.au/national-affairs/health/doctors-fees-real-villain-for-health-insurance-funds/news-story/998de470b02729bdb797c8d09630969a

6   https://www.pc.gov.au/inquiries/completed/productivity-review/report/2-healthier-australians

7   http://health.gov.au/internet/main/publishing.nsf/Content/Quarterly-Medicare-Statistics

8   Jeremy Sammut, Fiscal Fiction: The Real Medicare Levy, Research Report 29, (Sydney: The Centre for Independent Studies, 2017).

Chapter 2

Integrated Care and Alternative Payment Models*

Jeremy Sammut

Not Even Half a Solution to Health Costs in Australia

Aspects of the Australian health system resemble a black hole. Many of the billions of dollars of the near 10% of total GDP expended annually on health is spent ineffectively and inefficiently because health services are not provided in a market environment that delivers the best value for money—all necessary care at the highest quality and least cost. The problems created by cost-ineffective health spending include not only the increasingly unaffordable cost of health to the nation, but also the fact that the sickest and often poorest patients can miss out on all the care they require.

Many health experts in Australia maintain that the financial sustainability of Medicare can be improved by expanding the provision of lower-cost, 'coordinated' primary care services that will prevent chronically-ill patients from requiring high-cost hospital services. 'Gaps' in the Medicare system for chronic disease care—defined as a lack of access to a full range of community-based, multidisciplinary, medical, nursing, and allied healthcare—are reputed to cause hundreds of thousands of 'potentially preventable' hospital admissions per annum at a cost of hundreds of millions of dollars to the health system.

The most problematic public policy ideas are those that seem intuitively correct. These ideas attract support because they appear to be soundly-based and to offer obvious answers to important policy problems. But the intuition

* First published as Medi-Value: health insurance and service innovation in Australia -implications for the future of Medicare, Research Report 14, (Sydney: The Centre for Independent Studies, 2016).

may well be wrong; there may, in fact, be little evidence to support the effectiveness of what seems to be an entirely plausible and purely common sense approach to policy making. These points apply to one of the most popular and perennially suggested health policy ideas.

At the December 2015 Council of Australian Government's (COAG) meeting, Victorian Premier Daniel Andrews presented his federal and state and territory government counterparts with what the media billed as a "dramatic health reform plan" that could save the health system up to $1.5 billion a year. The Premier's proposal was to hire a new kind of publicly-employed health worker, a "care coordinator", whose role would be to work with chronically ill patients to ensure they have "coordinated patient care plans." The rationale for the proposal was that many thousands of chronically ill patients end up being admitted to hospitals each year because their conditions are not properly monitored, because they are not properly medicated, and because they do not access the full range of medical care from health professionals including nurses, podiatrists, and physiotherapists that can help them stay well and out of hospital. The care coordinators could remedy these defects, as well as fix defective communication between state-funded public hospitals and federally-funded GPs, pharmacists and allied health professionals, which was claimed to be a key driver of the 285,000 hospital admissions each year, or 10% of total annual national admissions, considered potentially avoidable. Mr Andrews argued health reform that addressed "the biggest problem in health at the moment" — by delivering different, better managed, and better organised chronic disease care — was a matter of ensuring government spending on the health system "is as efficient and effective as it possibly can be."[1]

In reality, there was little that was new in the proposals. Health experts and stakeholder groups routinely suggest that Medicare can be re-established on more sustainable fiscal and clinical foundations by re-orientating the system away from an over-reliance on very expensive hospital-based health services and by expanding the provision of lower-cost, 'community-based' primary healthcare services. This approach to "restructuring our health system to improve the effectiveness of primary care" is commonly said to be "about rational health economics", as this kind of "innovative healthcare reform" is based on "a very strong evidence base" and will result in "far fewer needing inpatient hospital care."[2]

The rationale for following this advice appears compelling. Hospitals are designed to provide acute bed-based care for patients when major illness strikes. The services that Australia's 698 public hospitals provide reflect the healthcare needs of the period when hospital systems were founded, between the mid-nineteenth through to the mid-twentieth century. But the times, and the health needs of the community, have changed. In the twenty-first century, the major health challenge is not simply to provide one-off treatments for acute illnesses. The major challenge is to provide ongoing care to address the rising burden of chronic illnesses — such as diabetes, heart disease, and respiratory disease — the onset of which is being driven on the one hand by the impact of a rapidly ageing population, and on the other hand by lifestyle factors principally related to obesity and unhealthy eating, drinking, and smoking habits.[3]

The argument goes that the failure to access non-hospital-based chronic disease services increases the demand for, and reliance on, hospital care. Because insufficient attention is paid to ensuring that chronic conditions are properly cared for in the community, many of these patients end up suffering acute episodes that require admission to hospital for treatment at substantial cost to taxpayers, and frequently at cost to private insurance funds as well, when patients have private cover and are admitted to private hospitals or privately to public hospitals.

But — as this chapter outlines — despite the apparent scope for new Medicare services to address the ever-escalating cost of hospital care, multiple Australian and international studies have shown that publicly-funded, bureaucratically-administered and centrally planned coordinated chronic disease programs have not achieved the anticipated reductions in use of hospital services. A 'top down', government-driven, primary care-focused health reform strategy is not even half a solution to the real problems associated with the high and rapidly increasing cost of healthcare in Australia.

Medicare's Structural Flaws

The problem of unnecessary or 'potentially preventable' hospital admissions by chronic patients also draws attention to the structural flaws in the complex funding and service arrangements that distinguish the Medicare system.

The federal government runs and funds the primary care part of Medicare. This is part of the function of overseeing the Medical Benefits Scheme (MBS), the principal function of which is to pay benefits to meet or assist in covering the cost of fees mainly for GP care, medical imaging and diagnostic services, and other specialist ambulatory and inpatient attendances and procedures on a fee-for-service, on-demand, and open-ended basis. The federal government also gives state and territory governments a fixed amount of money each year to partially fund the operation of public hospitals. Federal hospital funding is provided on condition that all Australians are entitled to receive 'free' public hospital care at point of access; but otherwise state and territory governments are responsible for hospital governance and administration.

Jurisdictional complexity—with the result being that neither level of government is solely accountable for the entire healthcare needs of patients—distorts responsibilities and incentives in ways that partially account for the service gaps (and ironically sometimes duplications, such as repeat tests and imaging services) for chronic patients. Medicare does not in all cases provide access to the full range of medical, pharmaceutical and allied healthcare that might ensure chronic conditions are properly managed to stop patients ending up in hospital.

Hence chronic disease services are often described as 'multi-disciplinary' or 'coordinated care'. These terms mean that in addition to the care of a general practitioner, a care coordinator, who may be a nurse, will monitor the condition and manage the care of the chronically ill to help patients navigate different parts of the health system successfully and receive all available care from a wide variety of allied health providers. Coordinated care also involves educating patients about their disease so they can better self-manage their condition and maintain their health. Self-management is particularly important if patients' conditions are complex and they have comorbidities that can cause complications and more frequent, longer, and costlier hospital stays. Hence, the cost-benefit rationale is that the additional costs associated with coordinated care compared to traditional GP care may be justified by both the improved health outcomes for patients and by the cost savings associated with avoiding the use of expensive hospital services.

The more targeted the approach, the more cost-effective the care coordination intervention is likely to be. This is because the population suffering chronic illness is not homogenous. Many people, even with multiple conditions, suffer relatively few adverse effects on their lives and use of health care with little impact on health costs. Standard GP care, combined with self-management, is sufficient for this patient group. It is highly complex patients, at severe risk of deteriorations and complications, who generate a disproportionate share of health costs, for whom more intensive assistance in the form of care coordination is appropriate—due to the real potential to relieve the burden otherwise imposed on scarce GP and hospital resources.[4]

The debate about chronic care has provoked a long-running 'blame game' between federal and state governments, as each would prefer that the other take responsibility and bear the cost of funding chronic disease services. State governments claim that closing the service gaps in the primary care system is a federal policy responsibility, and blame the persistence of the problem on federal government inertia. This seems fair enough, especially when the federal government can be said to foot part of the resulting financial burden, and is ultimately paying more in health grants to the states than it ought in order to fund otherwise preventable hospital admissions. Yet it could be said that state governments act equally irrationally, and that if there are cheaper and better ways to treat chronic disease in the community, they should just do it. Indeed, states do operate, on a piece-meal basis, a range of community-based programs with a focus on management of chronic disease. But despite the promised savings on the cost of hospital care, finding the additional resources to fund comprehensive chronic care services, amid limited budgets and competing priorities, is something neither level of government has proven capable of doing.

Action by either level of government has also been stymied by a common problem. Despite the widespread belief that existing funding is not being used optimally to meet the health needs of the community – that is the approximately $20 billion and $40 billion of taxpayer's money spent annually on Medicare-funded primary care and hospital care respectively - both federal and state governments have been unwilling to reallocate resources away from existing medical services or hospital services respectively. The reason for this is health politics: such action would be highly likely to generate significant opposition from affected provider groups, especially from general practitioners and hospital-based specialists whose current professional lives and incomes depend on the maintenance of the Medicare status quo. This includes the ability of specialists to admit privately-insured patients to public hospitals for treatment, and to thereby, in effect, use publicly-funded hospital infrastructure to operate private, fee-for-service medical business at considerable (and opaque) cost to taxpayers (see below).[5]

The bottom line, and political reality, is that due to the complex division of health responsibilities between the federal and state and territory governments under Australia's federation, neither level of government has been willing to address the real chronic condition in the Australian health system. This is a structural problem that means that Medicare is not a 'health system' per se, but primarily functions as a series of provider-oriented payment mechanisms for separate sets of non-hospital and hospital-based services. Medicare does not operate as a comprehensive health insurance and risk-management system that offers patients all necessary and beneficial care, no matter the setting or provider. Since no single funder is solely accountable for the entire healthcare needs of patients, and since providers of health services do not share full financial risk for all the health costs of patients either, neither funders nor providers have authority or sufficient financial incentives to ensure health resources are used as efficiently as possible to ensure patients receive the most appropriate and cost effective care and do not fall through the cracks.[6]

It must be noted, however, that the gaps in Medicare persist despite recent federal initiatives to improve access to chronic care services. Since 2005, MBS payments for chronic disease management have been available to doctors and allied health practitioners, at a cost to the federal budget now approaching $1 billion annually. It is highly likely that some chronic patients have received improved quality of care as a result.[7] But the addition of GP Management Plan (GPMP) and Team Care (TCA) items to the MBS is unlikely to have proved cost effective, due to the untargeted nature of these programs. Patients with low-level chronic illness, along with other consumers with no chronic disease at all who simply want to use subsidised allied health services, receive the same level of access as highly-complex patients. Hence there is evidence—according to the former head of the Medicare watch-dog, the Professional Services Review—that the writing of boilerplate GPMPs and TCAs for patients irrespective of clinical need has become a lucrative way of maximising the incomes of some practices. Likewise, adding allied health services to the MBS may have satisfied the professional aspirations, and enhanced the incomes, of physiotherapists and psychologists, but the creation of a new layer of services has had little observable effect on the quality and outcomes of chronic care in terms of realising the promised overall impact on health costs.[8]

This raises a further question: even if Australian governments find more money for chronic disease programs, will these new services actually work? In the perpetual push to fix what appears to be so obvious a defect as the chronic care gaps in Medicare, the lack of evidence demonstrating the effectiveness of publicly-funded and administered chronic disease programs is overlooked. Worse is that innovative patient-centred rather than provider-centric approaches, that might better address the chronic care gaps in the system and also achieve the system changes required to address Medicare's underlying structural problems and inefficiencies, do not receive the consideration they deserve.

Déjà Vu All Over Again – Primary Healthcare Debate 2007-2016

Abbott-Turnbull Primary Healthcare Policy

The current Federal Coalition Government, under the leadership of former Prime Minister Tony Abbott and now under Prime Minister Malcolm Turnbull, has embraced the idea of enhanced chronic care as a major feature of its health reform agenda. This embrace occurred mid-stream, as it were, during the government's first term, and the context requires explanation.

After winning the 2013 election on a platform of pledging to repair the budget deficit, the Abbott government announced that as a savings measure it would introduce a $7 compulsory patient co-payment for Medicare-funded GP and select medical services. The co-payment was designed to apply to services that formerly had been 'bulk billed'—which, that is, were paid for entirely by the benefit received by doctors under the MBS with no out-of-pocket charges being incurred by consumers. Due to the unpopularity of the new savings measure, and in response to a vigorous anti-co-payment campaign led by the implacable AMA, this policy was withdrawn in early 2015 after it was clear that it would not pass in the Senate due to lack of cross-bench support.

Following a change of portfolio, the new Health Minister, Sussan Ley, set about reconstructing the Coalition's health policy. This amounted to conducting a national listening tour in fulfillment of her pledge to consult more widely with health professionals, thereby addressing a complaint of the AMA that the co-payment had been sprung on doctors without warning. The government's demand-side rationale for a mandatory co-payment was that consumption of fee-for-service, bulk billed medical services at zero prices inevitably resulted in over-servicing. The new supply-side approach to tackling the problem of waste in the health system took the form of the commissioning of a number of reviews under the banner of 'Healthier Medicare' initiative.

The Medicare Benefits Schedule Review Taskforce was charged with the job of 'modernising' the MBS. This amounts to seeking to eliminate waste by subjecting all the services funded through the MBS to evidence-based assessment to ensure that Medicare funding is delivering quality and value in the form of the best patient outcomes possible for the health dollars expended. In announcing the MBS review, Ms Ley went to great lengths to stress that the broader reform objective was not simply to de-fund low-value, out-of-date or unsafe services for the sake of budget repair, but rather to free up resources that could be better and more sustainably redeployed to meet the healthcare needs of the community. "Any reform would need to have a core focus on delivering better patient outcomes," she said. For what the government had learned, through the minister's wide-ranging consultations with health professionals and consumers, was that Medicare urgently needed to be modernised to assist patients and practitioners better manage chronic illness.[9]

Clarifying that the government's policy was about health (hence the 'Healthier Medicare' moniker) not budget savings, was the purpose of the second expert-led review that was also commissioned. The Primary Health Care Advisory Group (PHCAG) was tasked with advising the government on the primary care reforms necessary to fill the chronic care gaps in Medicare. Allied to the objectives of the MBS review, the PHCAG also identified that the problem with the current fee-for-service MBS system was that it "largely links payment to an interaction between a doctor and patient" and rewards "episodic rather than coordinated, multidisciplinary care" involving a number of different health practitioners.[10] The PHCAG also identified that the reform challenge was to ensure the sustainability of the health system by ensuring resource allocation was efficient, and ensuring "the most effective use of existing primary healthcare funding to appropriately target and support people with chronic and complex health conditions."[11]

The Coalition's embrace of primary care reform filled its post-co-payment health policy void in a dual sense. The Abbott Government, also in pursuit of budget repair, had reneged on the hospital funding agreement struck by the Gillard Government in 2011, and had reduced the future level of federal health funding the states and territories would receive.[12] Promising to do 'something' about chronic care represented an attempt to make up for the funding shortfall by achieving savings to state hospital budgets by addressing the problem of potentially avoidable hospital admissions.

In early April 2016, the Turnbull government released its pre-election health policy proposals. The Abbott government's 'cuts' to hospital funding would be reversed, but for only four years until 2020, at an additional estimated cost of $2.9 billion.[13] At the subsequent COAG meeting, all jurisdictions agreed to continue to take action to reduce avoidable hospital admission—including the federal government through primary care reform.[14] Unveiled on the eve of COAG was a new federal 'Healthier Medicare' program—a $20 million trial ahead of a national rollout that aspires to enrol initially 65,000 chronic patients across 200 GP practices in a 'Health Care Home' with capitation funding for primary care service and coordination costs provided on a quarterly basis.[15]

Rudd-Gillard Primary Healthcare Policy

Yet the Coalition's approach to primary healthcare reform is largely reminiscent of the approach taken by its predecessor Labor Government. Before the 2007 federal election, the then leader of the opposition, Kevin Rudd, promised to "end the blame game" over health. In early 2008, as Prime Minister, Mr Rudd appointed a 10-member expert National Health and Hospitals Reform Commission (NHHRC) to review the health system and advise on the long-term reforms required to address the major health challenges of the twenty-first century. After conducting extensive consultations with health professionals and consumers, the 15-month NHHRC review culminated with release of its final report in July 2009. The 300-page A Healthier Future for All Australians made over 100 recommendations, but its major findings focused on the need for primary care reform.[16]

To consult the NHHRC report is to learn that the Coalition's Healthier Medicare initiative is traversing exactly the same ground. Like the PHCAG,[17] the NHHRC argued that the chief systemic barrier to better outcomes was the fragmentation of health services owing to the limitations of the MBS and the federal-state split in health responsibilities, which meant that patients with chronic conditions often received un-coordinated care and did not receive all the services they needed from a range of the health professionals.

Hence, the major reform challenge, and the way to end the blame game, was to find ways to improve access to Medicare-funded (i.e. federal government-funded) coordinated, multidisciplinary primary care to prevent avoidable hospital admissions.[18]

Like the PHCAG,[19] the NHHRC has already flagged that effective primary care reform may require changes to the existing Medicare fee-for-service funding arrangements and the introduction of payment models better suited to the requirements of longer-term, 'team-based' care. This included ideas such as requiring chronic patients to enrol with a primary care 'home', which would receive capitation funding—a fixed or block amount of funding per enrolled patient—to support the coordination and provision of primary care services across the spectrum.[20] The idea of a 'Health Care Home' was the major recommendation of the final report of the PHCAG,[21] and is now the Turnbull government's official primary healthcare policy in the shape of the Healthier Medicare program.[22]

The NHHRC maintained that the major health reform challenge was to improve health outcomes and health system sustainability by changing how and where health funding was spent; shifting away from a hospital-centric system required "evidence-based investment in strengthened primary healthcare services."[23] The problem, however, was that the evidence-base surveyed as part of the NHHRC process, did not support the claims made about the effectiveness of coordinated primary care.

Evidence-Based Policy—Or A Policy Looking for an Evidence-Base?

The idea of reorienting the health system around strengthened primary care services has been in vogue since at least the 1990s. To test the efficacy and build the evidence-base for this approach, the federal health department established the Australian Coordinated Care Trials. Funding from existing state and commonwealth health programs was 'pooled' and reallocated to nine community-based 'fundholding' organisations in six states and territories in order to support the provision of multidisciplinary care. The results of the trials were counter-intuitive.[24]

In general, the evaluation of the trials published in 2002 found that they had not improved health outcomes among participants and that most programs operated at a loss.[25] For example, one of the trials conducted in the northern suburbs of Melbourne coordinated the care of a trial group of elderly and chronically ill patients aged 75. But this was found to have produced no significant reduction in hospital use, compared to a control group that continued to receive their usual level of care from their GP.[26] The South Australian 'Health Plus' trial was partly successful and achieved some improvement in patient outcomes. Yet even in this trial—one of only three to register a significant reduction in hospital admissions—the savings on hospital costs were not sufficient to cover the higher costs of coordination.[27]

Commenting on the results in the Medical Journal of Australia, Adrian Esterman and David Ben-Tovim explained the trials showed the essential premise that better coordination reduces hospitalisations is misguided. It may be that lack of coordination in a complex care system operates as a functioning rationing system, so better care coordination reveals unmet needs rather than resolving them.[28]

This conclusion was consistent with the overwhelming bulk of the research assessing the results of coordinated care programs.[29] Rather than reduce use of hospitals by preventing avoidable admissions, a range of studies and evaluations has suggested that lack of coordination does indeed act as rationing device, whereby insufficient access to primary care prevents referral to hospital care. Hence a significant effect of coordination that has been observed is to actually increase use of hospitals by uncovering unmet need and ensuring patients (particularly low socio-economic status patients who lack the means or knowledge to coordinate their own care) receive all beneficial hospital care.[30] (Box 1)

That patients who receive coordinated care can receive all beneficial primary and hospital care is clearly a good outcome for patients. Nevertheless, this contradicts the central claims that have been made about its supposed effects on use of health services.[31] The evidence that coordinated care programs haven't delivered the foretold reduction in hospital admissions was evaluated by the discussion paper written by Professor Leonie Segal, which was commissioned by the NHHRC to supposedly inform its work. The summary of the evidence compiled by Segal was telling:

> Whilst it has also been postulated that high quality primary care will reduce the use and cost of hospital services by substituting for less appropriate or more expensive tertiary inpatient or emergency department care and improving the quality of chronic disease management and lowering rates of disease progression and complications the evidence here is equivocal. Some success in small scale intervention trials is observed, but this is not necessarily translated into larger population based interventions. While reasons can be posited as to why the 'expected reduction' in hospital admission did not occur, it is plausible that high quality primary care may be additive to, rather than a replacement for hospital care. In any case, 'ambulatory care sensitive' admissions (potentially avoidable through high quality primary care), for diabetes complications, COPD etc. have been estimated to account for only 10% of hospital admissions. Reform of primary care should be justified in terms of its impact on health and wellbeing and equity, rather than presumed 'cost savings.'[32]

These findings—that coordinated care programs offer an additional layer of service for no cost-benefit (as opposed to health outcome) return—are also consistent with the 2012 report by the United States Congressional Budget Office (CBO), which examined the effectiveness of chronic care programs implemented by the US federal government over the previous two decades.[33] The report examined 34 nurse-led care coordination 'demonstration projects' that aimed to educate patients, encourage compliance with self-care regimes, and track and target appropriate clinical services. In the words of America healthcare expert, John Goodman, the CBO found that on average these projects had had "little or no effect on hospital admissions" and that nearly every project's impact on "spending was either unchanged or increased relative to the spending that would have occurred in the absence of the program."[34]

Box 1. A Rationing Device

- In 2003, for example, the UK government commissioned a pilot coordinated care program. Practice nurses conducted comprehensive geriatric assessments of elderly patients not in regular contact with general practice services, designed individual care plans, and undertook follow-up monitoring.

- The evaluation of the pilot program found that "case management had no significant impact on rates of emergency admission, bed days, or mortality in high risk cohorts." The evaluation suggested that while better coordination might avoid hospitalisations in individual cases, overall, instead of reducing admissions in the wider population, improved access to coordinated primary care uncovered new cases requiring hospitalisation.[35]

- In 2004, the New Zealand Ministry of Health introduced a new scheme to coordinate the care of chronic disease patients. The 'Care Plus' program allocated extra funding to New Zealand's eighty-one publicly funded Primary Health Organisations. This entitled the chronically ill to receive reduced-cost nurse or doctor visits, care planning, and self-management support.

- The independent evaluation found that the program had improved the care of Care Plus patients, but had led to higher, not lower, utilisation of medical services. In this case, when coordinated care was translated from the trial to the real world, it led to consultation rates increasing by four visits per annum on average. This led to hospital admissions rising by 40%, an outcome attributed to better monitoring of chronically ill patients' conditions.[36]

"Did Not Occur"—Top Down, Not Bottom Up

"So why is none of this working?" asks Goodman. The reasons seem hard to fathom. Many severely chronically ill people are socially disadvantaged and struggle for personal and financial reasons to access all beneficial services and comply with appropriate treatment regimes. There appears to be much scope for new services to succeed and yet the expected reductions in hospital use have not happened.

It is plausible that the failure of chronic care programs to yield the promised savings and to demonstrate their cost-effectiveness is due to a dual effect. The uncovering of unmet need among patients formerly receiving inadequate care has 'compromised' the initial results of the trials. If this is a one-off effect—which is yet to be demonstrated, particularly for elderly chronic disease patients—properly targeted care coordination could demonstrate its effectiveness over a longer time-frame as the benefits of secondary prevention and earlier intervention, particularly enhanced self-management, achieve reductions in the cost of care and absorb care coordination costs. It is also reasonable to suggest that the additional cost of coordination can be justified by discovering unmet need and improving health outcomes at a higher cost. Despite how inherently worthy such an outcome is, this is not the policy proposition that drives the coordinated care debate—which is that the investment in quality primary care will deliver a lower cost, and more cost-effective health system by reducing 'preventable hospital admissions'.

A recent report by the Grattan Institute restated the case for "much greater investment in supporting service development and innovation in primary care." The report underlined the gaps in the existing system for chronic care that were said to be a driver of higher costs, and reasoned that improving the management and quality of primary care would improve clinical outcomes and yield savings. It identified that the existing $1.7 billion in total government funding on chronic disease management was not effective, principally due to the funding having been grafted onto the existing Medicare fee-for-service system. Even the Practice Service and Incentive Program introduced in the 1990s—which was intended to supplement the fee-for-service system and standardise best practice chronic care—has had limited uptake by GPs, limited patient enrolment, and thus limited overall effectiveness. The authors argued that "[e]vidence from around the world suggests that much greater emphasis needs to be placed on service coordination and integration with chronic disease." This is not the same thing as arguing the international evidence shows chronic care 'innovation' had achieved the promised results. The authors therefore admitted the evidence is limited with respect to what works, given the evidence-base primarily consists of the 'promising' results of some small scale studies. They also, however, rightly identified that the major barrier to large-scale and genuine innovation is the difficulty involved in achieving comprehensive structural reform of the existing health systems. The Grattan Institute may hereby have identified the problem, but not the solution. The report's major recommendation is to call for a 'system redesign' to resolve jurisdictional complexities in the split federal-state health system in Australia by creating a new layer of public sector bureaucracy: region-based health agencies responsible for coordinating and integrating care, for fostering innovation including in payment mechanisms, and for setting targets and measuring outcomes.[37]

The reform model recommended by Grattan—which can be described as a top-down approach to implementing 'public sector managed care'—actually points to another possible answer to the chronic care puzzle. This concerns not simply the clinical issues relevant to chronic care per se, but rather the method or means of production behind the delivery of these services. Goodman argues that expecting a public health bureaucracy to centrally-plan a supposedly innovative program is demonstrably flawed in conception and execution. This approach fails because the proper roles that ought to be played by buyers and sellers of goods and services are confused in bureaucratic health systems. "Successful innovations are produced by entrepreneurs, challenging conventional thinking—not by bureaucrats trying to implement conventional thinking." In the case of chronic care services, "buyers of a product (i.e. health bureaucrats) are trying to tell the sellers how to efficiently produce it".[38] In efficient markets, real innovation is not driven from the top down by buyers telling sellers what to do, but is generated from the bottom up by entrepreneurs operating in competitive environments who discover new, better, and lower cost ways to deliver services to cost-conscious buyers—who are free to choose between competing providers based on quality and price. (Box 2)

Another top-down approach to improving the quality of clinical care, particularly for chronic disease, is pay-for-performance (P4P) mechanisms that use financial incentives to encourage healthcare providers to meet pre-established performance targets. These schemes can range from reward payments for complying with evidence-based 'best practice' guidelines, to conditional payments for attaining particular outcomes, to no payment for poor results. Yet the limited evidence gathered from evaluations of P4P schemes is not promising. A 2011 systematic review of P4P chronic care programs by de Bruin and others found some positive effects on healthcare quality, as in compliance with the service targets that had to be hit to trigger the financial rewards. But the evaluations contained no evidence about the effects on healthcare costs.[39] Likewise, two 2011 Cochrane reviews of P4P schemes similarly found that while processes of care had been improved, there was no evidence concerning patient outcomes, and such measures (along with the consequent impact on health costs) were rarely even included in the evaluations.[40]

Box 2. The Dedicated Person Problem—Times Two

- Goodman identifies another related problem with the bureaucratic production of chronic services: 'promising trials' (not only in health but in many areas of government activity in general) tend to fail because they do not scale.

- Even successful trials frequently fail to translate in the real world because they strike up against the 'dedicated person problem'.

- Firstly, a trial may have been successful due to the knowledge, expertise, and commitment of those who planned and staffed it. The same levels of skill and dedication are unlikely to be found throughout the workforce employed under a full-scale program.

- Secondly, a chronic care trial may have been successful because the patients who participated were especially motivated to improve their conditions, and hence are unlike the de-motivated patients who are the real targets of these programs, and who may well have dropped out of the trial and thus distorted the results.[41]

- For example, the UK 'Expert Patients Programme' had limited uptake and therefore limited success and applicability. A national evaluation published in 2007 found "some reductions in costs of hospital use," but warned that the results should be treated with caution because they "are pertinent to people who volunteer to go on such a course and not those with long-term conditions generally."[42]

The apparent design flaws in the evaluations are, in truth, a product of the inherent limitations of P4P schemes. By their very nature, these programs reward compliance with care processes that are simpler to measure rather than rewarding outcomes that are difficult to measure. It is particularly difficult to measure and reward the long-term impact on chronic disease, as it is hard to attribute the effect to a service provided at a point in the past, and when the determinants of patient well-being may lie outside reach of clinical services. Hence, in reality, P4P schemes can end up amounting to just another form of rules-based, centrally-planned fee-for-service payments.[43]

This seems to have been the result of the system-wide P4P scheme introduced in the UK. Under the UK National Health Scheme (NHS), GPs are funded by 'blended' payments combining elements of capitation, fee-for-service and performance payments. A key aim of the Quality and Outcomes Framework (QOF) introduced in 2004 was to improve the quality of primary care by encouraging GPs to better manage and coordinate the care of chronic patients to avoid hospitalisation. Hence, up to a quarter of GP income was at risk if quality targets for chronic care were not met. But about half of those targets concerned clinical process, and most of the remainder concerned administrative process and recording patient experience. Few targets, and only a small proportion of reward payments, were linked to patient outcomes.[44]

As would be expected, the things that were rewarded were the things that were done. The QOF was found to have improved care processes and quality to the extent of GP practices reorganising and systematising how they managed chronic patients. But there is no evidence that compliance with 'tick a box' process measures has had a positive impact on patient outcomes, particularly with respect to use of hospitals. Nor, therefore, could it be established that the QOF was cost-effective and that the additional cost reduced the total health cost across the system.[45]

Moreover, the scheme appears to have been gamed, created perverse incentives, and had unintended consequences. Most providers rapidly attained the targets to significantly boost GP practice incomes, but at the expense of neglecting other areas of patient care not subject to financial incentives.[46] There are also concerns that the link between income and the rigid framework led to rote practice and prevented the development of tailored services that suit the complex needs of local populations. In other words, the top-down approach to mandating so-called quality has actually operated as a barrier impeding genuine innovation.[47]

This has implications for the Healthier Medicare program that raise concerns. The Turnbull government's plan to create 'Health Care Homes' has some attractive features. The positives include the use of risk stratification to identify, and target for enrolment, the most high-risk chronic disease sufferers. Yet enrolment is voluntary, which begs the question whether patients unmotivated enough to find a 'home' themselves will bother to participate and stick with the program. Also positive are promises of improved collection of data, information sharing between services, and development of performance and outcome measures. Yet the program will essentially be structured around the application of evidence-based clinical guidelines, and as such represents a top-down approach rather than a leap into the discovery process that generates true innovation. The introduction of capitation payment is a significant development, and will create additional flexibility in terms of the potential access to a broader range of primary care services and coordination services. But will the 'Health Care Homes' be a home in name only? Both the PHCAG final report and the details released by the governments suggest a major focus will be on working to resolve jurisdictional complexities. By some undefined process, the herculean task of unscrambling the federal-state health split is anticipated in order to establish local care pathways for enrolled patients, which will also integrate primary and secondary care. This is despite the fact that the 'Health Care Homes' will have financial control only over the provision of out-of-hospital care. Hence the program is highly likely to struggle to achieve its objective of effectively coordinating, in an innovative fashion, all the care patients require across the spectrum, as Health Care Homes will instead have to rely on existing referral and treatment options for in-hospital services.[48]

Implications for Australian Health Reform

The insights that can be gained from the US and UK public health system's experiments in chronic care are important to the Australian health reform debate. Most of the proposals for enhanced primary care services in Australia plan on using the public health bureaucracy to implement 'innovative' chronic care, as the recent Grattan Institute report demonstrates. Yet the evidence is clear: all indications are that the envisaged public sector managed care reform options—which either entail getting the federal health department to fund, state health departments to fund, or the 'pooling' of federal and state funding to pay for, coordinated chronic disease programs—are destined to disappoint in terms of yielding the much-hyped and promised cost savings.

Expecting federal, state, or even new region-based joint federal-state health agencies[49] to act as purchasers of packages of chronic care services tailored to patient's needs, will inevitably replicate the design faults inherent in bureaucratic programs. The problem is that public sector bureaucracies need to know what they are buying and paying for before they commit taxpayer's money to particular programs. This is why government programs are designed from the top down, and consist of rules-based, centrally-administered protocols that dictate all the things providers must do. Providers do what the bureaucracies are willing to pay for; compliance stymies real innovation, and this explains why many public programs are ineffective. Governments under these inflexible command-and-control arrangements end up paying for things they know will be done, rather than paying for what works.

These problems are compounded by the culture of the public health system, given its essential nature as a payment system for a set of pre-determined clinical services. Program funding for care coordination, particularly if public sector employed and unionised nurses are funded to fulfil this task, will extend the provider-based nature of the public health system into the chronic care arena. Because the political economy of the public health system creates powerful vested interests, withdrawing program funding will be very difficult, even if the new chronic care services prove ineffective—which is highly likely if the nursing profession's declared ambition to secure community-based clinical roles for nurses is satisfied under the rubric of chronic care.[50]

Goodman cites an example of a successful chronic care program. An entrepreneurial doctor in New Jersey understood that healthcare costs could be lowered by targeting high-cost chronic disease patients who made frequent use of health and hospital services. The service he developed, the 'Camden Coalition', does more than simply provide conventional medical care. Patients are offered what really amounted to social work for those with a range of social problems (such as homelessness and drug abuse) that exacerbated their illness and made it difficult to properly manage their health conditions. Despite the savings generated to the public health system, the Camden Coalition has to rely solely on private philanthropy to fund its activities. This is because the top-down, command-and-control US public health system does not pay for this kind of unconventional medico-social work, despite it working. Attempts to secure public funding ran up against bureaucratic obstacles in government agencies used to dictating the services providers must supply and the amount they will pay based on a set of protocols.[51]

The lesson is that if innovation is to flourish, it needs to be nurtured by a real market in which there are real buyers and real sellers of health services. This is a challenging lesson because it stands much of the existing health economy on its head. Expecting health bureaucracies to centrally plan supposedly innovative programs is a demonstrably flawed approach. Real innovation is not driven from the top down, by paying providers to comply with clinical protocols and carry out prescribed tasks at a set funding 'price' as is, in essence, the design of the government driven Healthier Medicare program. Real innovation speaks of a more dynamic, competitive and contestable environment that will enable innovative ways of providing health services to be generated from the bottom up. Entrepreneurial providers that deliver cost-effective, patient-centred healthcare need to be able to thrive and be rewarded for discovering what works to increase efficiency and lower costs, by being able to sell that value proposition to purchasers who care about price, quality, and effectiveness.[52]

International Experience

Literature discussing the failure of top-down primary care reform efforts reveals additional support for reconfiguring how healthcare is funded as a first step towards improving the quality and efficiency of health services. For healthcare to be considered truly coordinated across the health system, it needs to span the divide between hospital and community-based settings. Existing primary care reform strategies struggle to bridge this divide due to the institutional and fee-for-service payment system legacies of established health systems, which foster inefficient practice and encourage over-servicing. Herein lies the purpose of recent initiatives, mainly by innovative private insurers in the United States, to develop integrated care and payment models to improve overall health system efficiency.[53]

Integrated care is fundamentally different to standard coordinated primary care programs.[54] Integrated payment models are designed to ensure that financial risk for both the hospital and non-hospital health costs of patients is shared with health service providers by combining traditional health funding streams into one bundled payment (which can be adjusted for risk factors). Providers who — in return for the specified payment — are contracted to deliver all the healthcare of patients out of an agreed global budget for a specified time period have a superior incentive to change traditional patterns of care, efficiently manage the care pathway and the full cycle of care of patients, and provide the most appropriate care in the lowest-cost setting. They thus have a financial incentive to focus on improving both performance and patient outcomes by discovering what actually works best — the optimal service mix, design, and structure — to keep patients out of hospital. While fee-for-service payments encourage over-servicing by rewarding providers based on the volume of services delivered, and capitation payment alone (for siloed primary or hospital services) can encourage providers to under-service and deny care to limit costs without improving outcomes, integrated payments incentivise providers to deliver the right amount and right type of care at the right time — or bear financial responsibility for the additional cost of inefficiency and adverse outcomes for patients.[55]

Compared to the lack of evidence to support existing approaches to primary care reform, making service providers financially accountable for quality and cost across the continuum of healthcare looms as the logical and clear-cut way to generate cost-effective service innovations from the bottom up.[56] Examples of promising improvements in quality, efficiency, and reductions in cost of care include the Gesundes Kinzigtal scheme in south-west Germany, where a health management company has contracted with the government insurer to provide—in partnership with a local physicians' network—both primary and hospital care for insured patients.[57] The 'Alzira model' developed in the Valencia region of Spain has similarly achieved positive results after the private operator of the local public hospital also assumed responsibility for the primary care. The private company made the integrated capitation contract work financially by both developing chronic disease programs and improving the productivity of the hospital.[58] Similar privatisation in other regions of Valencia has reputedly reduced costs by 25% through use of capitation funding and by permitting competition between hospitals.[59]

Integrated payments models are also known as "value-based contracting."[60] This is apt because the term more accurately describes the financial incentives in play, which allow providers to share in the value they create by achieving efficiencies, particularly by reducing use of hospitals.

To put it bluntly, traditional health systems take large sums of health dollars off the table through payment systems that reward inefficient practice and over-use of services. Integrated payment models put that money back on the table, and give providers a financial incentive to gain a share of that money according to the value they can add to the system for insurers by eliminating waste and by achieving cost-saving improvements. Providers who create value by better managing the cost of care below the value of the service contract are rewarded by being able to retain (all or part of) the savings achieved by making more efficient overall use of health system resources.[61]

Sharing financial risk with providers through value-based contacting may require the insurance side of public health systems to be transformed from simple funding or payment mechanisms into authentic insurance risk-management systems. Literature canvassing the failure of existing approaches to health reform outlines that this initial transformation is a step towards addressing the problem of funding and institutional silos across primary care and hospital sectors, and the resulting system inefficiencies. Hence Charlesworth, Davies and Dixon argued in their review of NHS payment reforms that real progress towards a more efficient integrated care and value-based contracting model would require substantial changes to the UK's taxpayer-funded public health system architecture, along the lines of that which has occurred in Netherlands, which in 2006 replaced its traditional Medicare-style public health system with a market-based system of publicly-funded insurance vouchers and competing private health insurance funds.[62]

The transformation of the insurance side of the Netherlands health system has led to experiments in new purchasing and payment arrangements. This includes pioneering development of 'episodic payments' for inpatient care, which bundle all the costs associated with a normal procedure, including the doctor's fee, into a single payment to a hospital. In combination with price contestability—the value of episodic payments is negotiated between insurers and hospitals—this has encouraged the development of more efficient specialist clinics that focus on treating particular conditions.[63]

In 2010, to further promote efficiency through enhanced care coordination, payments for chronic disease (diabetes, chronic obstructive pulmonary disease, vascular risk management) care were bundled together into a single contestable fee. Region-based 'care groups' (usually owned by GPs) have contracted with insurers to provide specific chronic disease services for patients—but only across primary settings. Not only was hospital care excluded from the disease-specific bundle (along with any general care required), but the generic services covered by the single fee (which included check-ups by practice nurses and sub-contracted allied healthcare by other providers) were centrally-determined by the national health department, complete with care protocols and aggregate quality targets and indicators.[64]

The Dutch 'innovations' more closely resemble the QOF in the UK, and thus seem to constitute a form of performance-based fee-for-service arrangement, rather than a truly integrated, outcomes-orientated, and value-based care and payment system. Unsurprisingly, an evaluation found that while processes of care had improved, the administrative burden was great, and large differences in price and performance not explained by differences in levels of care were are also found. This could be attributed not only to the lack of sufficient financial incentives to generate efficiencies, but also to lack of sufficient provider competition within regions dominated by a single care group.[65]

Despite the changes to health insurance architecture, the Netherlands appears to have persisted with a top-down approach to primary health reform. This suggests that even transforming the insurance side of health economy is not enough to transform service provision if this does not lead to sharing financial risk with truly integrated and financially accountable providers. The importance of integrating financial risk with service delivery is highlighted by one of the best-known but often misrepresented examples of fully integrated and accountable care health management and service provision: Kaiser Permanente.

Kaiser Permanente—Managing Care, Risk, & Utilisation

The managed care regimes pioneered in the United States by Health Maintenance Organisations (HMOs), are often cited in support of the promised benefits of coordinated primary care.[66] The cost-effective, high-quality model of care developed by the California HMO Kaiser Permanente is an especially popular example, but its lessons are selectively cited. One of the key lessons is to recommend allowing insurers and providers to share financial risk for member's healthcare costs.

Kaiser Permanente attracted renewed international attention following the publication in 2002 of a study that compared its performance against the British NHS. It was found that Kaiser achieved better performance outcomes at a lower cost: far superior access to specialist and tertiary treatment compared to the much longer waiting times for specialist and hospital treatment in the NHS. The key finding was that "age adjusted rates of use of hospital services in Kaiser were one third of those in the NHS."[67]

Due to the competitive nature of the US health market, HMOs aim to provide almost immediate access to medical care, and they accomplish this by managing the care of patients to ensure all medical services are provided in the most appropriate, efficient, and cost-effective setting. HMOs like Kaiser Permanente take a cost- and access-conscious approach to managed care because they have to compete with other HMOs for the custom of health insurance buyers (mainly governments and employers) who bargain hard on price. They also have to compete against strict indemnity insurance rivals, and thus satisfy individual members, who are demanding customers and are free to move between HMOs if dissatisfied. Competition and choice create the incentive to keep costs low while being responsive to patient demand.

The Kaiser in-house model of service delivery is different to the medical network model — which integrates independent providers into a coordinated care system — discussed in the sections above and below. Kaiser operates its own community-based health centres that employ physician assistants and nurses to provide patient care, as well as accredited doctors who are able to perform quite complex procedures to free up other specialists for more serious cases. Kaiser, like other HMOs in the US, also identifies high-risk chronic disease patients and offers coordinated chronic disease programs led by practice nurses. Kaiser's salaried employees across the health professions, including doctors, are also committed to the philosophy of delivering team-based multidisciplinary care.[68]

The 2002 study found that compared with NHS patients: "Kaiser patients are far more likely to receive appropriate treatment and intervention for diabetes and heart disease."[69] This might appear to suggest that Kaiser's lower frequency of hospital admission can be attributed to the resources-focused enhanced primary care services. However, this overlooks a 2004 study by Firemen and others, which found that Kaiser Permanente's programs, while improving the quality of patient care, did not decrease costs as expected. Higher spending on better-coordinated primary care had not produced the predicted cost savings on reduced hospital admissions—which "did not happen, despite increased use of effective medications and improved risk-factor control"—to offset the substantially higher cost of providing higher quality primary care.[70]

Moreover, the 2002 study actually found that what overwhelmingly accounted for "the nearly four times the number of acute bed days per 1000 population per year in the NHS than in Kaiser" was efficient use of expensive hospital beds. The reason for Kaiser delivering more care at lower cost was, as the study outlined, the striking difference "in the management of admissions and length of stays," which meant that "Kaiser members spend one third of the time in hospital compared with NHS patients."[71]

In other words, hospital beds were used more intensively or not used at all, due to rigorous management of hospital admissions and discharge procedures and because by overcoming the traditional institutional divide between primary and hospital care, Kaiser can treat more patients for more conditions in its lower cost community-based health centres. This—plus having two to three times the number of specialists the NHS does—was why "Kaiser can provide more and better paid specialists and perform more medical interventions with much shorter waiting times than the NHS for roughly the same per capita cost." The study also indicated that this was why Kaiser could afford the additional costs of superior-quality nurse-led chronic disease care.[72]

Accountable Quality Contracts in Massachusetts

There is a perception that the lessons of Kaiser Permanente have limited applicability to other health systems. This is because the outcomes Kaiser achieves are said to reflect the unique features of its in-house provision of care, including the internal culture of its staff (especially the willingness of doctors to work for salary as part of medical teams) which has taken decades to develop.

Yet there is emerging evidence that American insurers –seeking to rein in the out-of-control cost of US healthcare - can achieve Kaiser-style results if they strike the right contractual relationship with integrated and financially accountable providers. This shows that insurers do not necessarily need to run their own in-house facilities to achieve the same results as Kaiser, but can outsource management of all aspects of patient care to health management companies. Health management companies can then create a medical network by sub-contracting service delivery to individual providers, while providing the infrastructure necessary to overcome fragmentation and manage or coordinate the care of patients by: investing in communication and electronic health record IT; monitoring service usage and outcomes; redesigns of care pathways; and operating targeted chronic disease programs. The best evidence of the potential impact the right financial incentives and financially accountable health service provision can have is the promising results of the pioneering development of 'shared-risk' contracts by Blue Cross Blue Shield of Massachusetts. Here, health management companies are providing Kaiser-style results by providing networks of otherwise separate healthcare providers with the leadership and management required to deliver integrated care.[73]

In 2009, Blue Cross Blue Shield initiated a new integrated payment program, the Alternative Quality Contract (AQC). Under the terms of the contract, health management companies agreed to manage the care of Blue Cross members in return for an annual risk-adjusted budget based on historic per-member spending. The 'global payment' covered the cost of care across the entire primary, specialist and hospital care continuum for a patient population for a specified period, combined with bonus payments for meeting specified quality indicators. All healthcare accessed by members, whether delivered by a provider belonging to the health management company's sub-contracted 'medical group' network or by a non-network provider, is funded from the medical group's budget. At the end of the year, total payments are reconciled with the budget, and any money left over is paid to the medical group company. ACQs are two-sided—or shared savings and shared risk—contracts. Part or full financial risk for exceeding the budget target is born by the medical groups on either 50% or 100% basis depending on the level of the risk accepted by the provider. By holding providers accountable for cost of care, Blue Cross's ambition across the five-year term of the contracts was to cut annual growth in healthcare spending in half.[74]

Under the ACQ, patients were enrolled with a medical group based on the affiliation of their doctor of choice. The group was thereafter responsible for managing their care by acting, in effect, as their medical home, or rather by creating a patient-centred 'medical neighbourhood'.[75] Alert to the need in a competitive insurance market to ensure members received excellent care, Blue Cross sought to ensure that medical groups did not skimp on services to reduce costs, by including in the contracts generous financial incentives (up to 10% of the global budget, 5% for primary care, 5% for hospital care) for high quality as measured by 64 process, outcome and patient experience indicators covering inpatient and outpatient care. Blue Cross does not just provide regular updates on group spending and service usage, including comparative data from other providers. In addition to the financial incentives, it also provides data and feedback on quality scores, practice variations, and other information that will assist medical groups to hit quality targets such as by ensuring patients receive chronic care management services. To drive cultural change, encourage teamwork, and build support for the objectives of the ACQ contract, groups used—or intended to introduce—bonuses for doctors, linked to quality improvements and efficient use of services.[76] Since 2011, ACQ contracts have linked quality to shared savings and losses, with higher quality scores entitling providers to larger savings and to smaller shares of budget overruns.[77]

However, ACQs are no standard pay-for-performance program, due to the way real financial accountability encourages innovations that improve financial performance. This was the key finding of the evaluation undertaken of the eight medical groups that signed the first contracts. The evaluators found, as might be expected, that the groups had implemented case management strategies that targeted high-cost 'frequent flyers'—members with multiple chronic diseases at risk of requiring expensive hospitalisations. This encompassed a range of initiatives that incorporated use of multidisciplinary coordinated care programs, but also included more intensive interventions with high risk patients—such as automatic contacting of discharged patients to ensure that discharge instructions were understood, medications were being taken, appropriate support services were engaged, and to monitor potential complications and side-effects. This also included home visits to monitor conditions and help with compliance with care plans. Some groups even employed their own clinicians to perform discharge planning, and placed case managers in hospital emergency departments to prevent unnecessary admission.[78] These efforts have been underpinned by investment in data management systems to improve both management of chronic care and clinician performance, and form part of overall efforts to increase efficiency of delivery systems by redesigning clinical and administrative processes.[79]

The evaluation found that ACQ groups achieved lower average growth in spending compared to other Blue Cross HMO providers. But even more significantly, this appears to have been due to rigorous management of hospital utilisation, more than due to successful management of chronic disease. These savings were found to be due to effective targeting of what was described as 'low-hanging fruit', or as having "accrued largely from shifts in services towards providers with lower outpatient facility fees."[80] To underline the point, the evaluation quoted one medical director's telling comments about the group's chief managed care objective: "What we really want to avoid is our patients receiving unnecessary care in the most expensive places in town." The focus on controlling hospital use was particularly important, in the words of the evaluators, because "in Massachusetts...nearly half of all hospital admissions are to high-cost teaching hospitals."[81]

Low-cost groups focused on utilisation review and referral management to direct patients to less expensive facilities and settings. This involved implementing procedures to monitor referrals and educate clinicians about the cost of sending patients to much more expensive services outside the group's network of preferred providers. Hence, some groups explored adding specialists to their networks as the cheaper way to provide faster access to care. Managing referrals and hospital utilisation was found to be the highest priority for many groups because of the considerable cost savings that could be made by preventing admission to high-cost major hospitals. One group chose to sub-contract half its business from one preferred hospital to a different provider not only because fees were lower, but also because it was willing to share in the group's goal of using medical resources efficiently and agreed to assist with care coordination by sharing medical records and "to return patients to outpatient settings as quickly as possible."[82]

The initial evaluation found that the savings achieved by reducing prices and utilisation had not recouped the additional cost of quality bonuses. A subsequent evaluation of the first four years found that medical groups achieved an average saving of 6.8% compared to what was being spent on the same patients prior to the introduction of the ACQ. Average spending by ACQ medical groups was also found to have grown by less, compared to control groups in other states. These promising financial results were cost-effective; that is, they were achieved without compromising quality, with the improvements in quality achieved by ACQ medical groups generally exceeding those recorded elsewhere in the United States. Furthermore, by the fourth year of the ACQ's operation, net savings were achieved that exceeded the cost of quality incentives. It was found that 60% of the savings were generated by reduced prices (directing patients to less expensive providers) and 40% by reduced utilisation of procedures, imaging and testing, successfully bending the cost curve down for both inpatient and outpatient spending for ACQ groups compared to the control.[83] (Figure 1)

Hospital Utilisation—Identifying the Problem and Solution

What do the lessons from US managed care regimes mean for health reform in Australia? Advocates of the Coalition's primary care-focused health reform agenda rightly argue that rising government health expenditure in Australia is being largely driven by the increasing cost of hospital care.[84] They also

Figure 1: Cost Savings in Blue Cross Shield ACQs

Unadjusted Spending in the 2009 Alternative Quality Contract (AQC) Cohort versus the Control Group, 2006–2012.

Panel A shows the total unadjusted spending. Panel B shows the results according to site of care (inpatient [IP] or outpatient [OP]) and type of claim (facility [Fac] or professional [Prof]). The control group comprised commercially insured enrollees in employer-sponsored plans across eight Northeastern states: Connecticut, Maine, New Hampshire, New Jersey, New York, Pennsylvania, Rhode Island, and Vermont. The vertical line at the start of 2009 indicates the start of the AQC period.

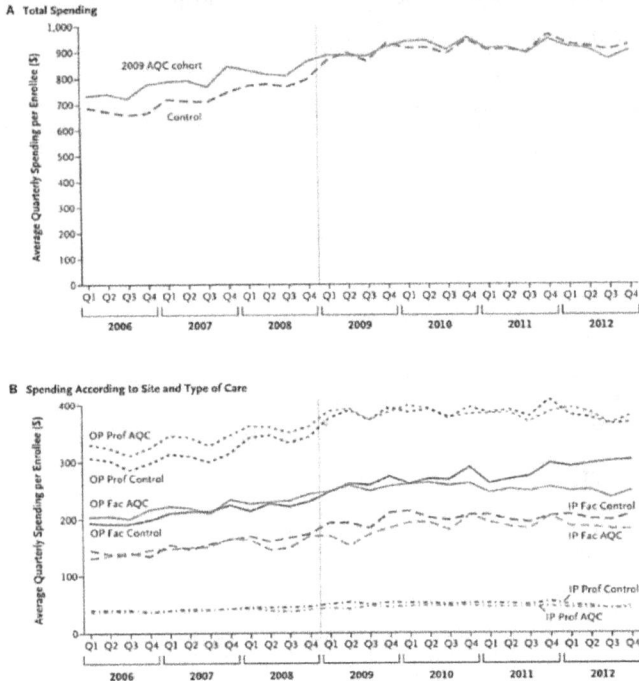

Source: Z. Song, et.al, "Changes in Health Care Spending and Quality 4 Years into Global Payment", New England Journal of Medicine, 371, 18, 2014.

point to the fact that acute hospital bed numbers in Australia remain at 3.8 per 1000 people, while comparable countries in the OECD have achieved a considerable reduction in bed numbers over the last decade. It is claimed that "the only way to reduce bed numbers sustainably is to keep people healthy" and this is said to require "innovative models" that will offer "integrated care outside of hospital to avoid hospitalising, particularly for chronic disease" — as is the intent of the government's Healthier Medicare initiative.[85]

2. Integrated Care and Alternative Payment Models

It is difficult to compare bed numbers across different countries and with different health systems, particularly given the geographical realities that dictate hospital bed provision in rural Australia. Nevertheless, there is strong evidence that Australia over-uses hospital care compared to other OECD nations. Australia has much higher acute hospital separations per person (0.41) and acute hospital bed days per person (2.36) than comparable countries such as the UK (0.27 and 0.57 respectively) and US (0.13 and 0.7 respectively).[86]

But does the high use of hospitals in Australia inexorably point to inadequate chronic care?[87] Not completely, given that 10% of admissions are classified as 'potentially preventable'. A likely explanation for high hospital usage compared to the UK is the much larger number of privately-owned hospital beds allied with much higher rates of strict-indemnity, fee-for-service private hospital insurance cover—which reward both hospital operators and specialists for the volume of services provided, and encourages both to ensure that hospital beds are filled. The characteristics of Australia's private health system that encourage supplier-induced demand are reinforced by the characteristics of Australia's public hospital system. Under the terms of their contracts, specialists working as either Visiting Medical Officers (VMOs) or Staff Specialists have the right to admit private patients to public hospitals. The ability to access publicly-funded hospital infrastructure has allowed specialists, in effect, to operate small businesses offering procedural care to privately insured patients at public expense. The enduring ability of specialists to access free public capital (in addition to their private hospital work) seems to have militated against any wholesale shift away from hospital-based care in favour of delivering specialist procedures in community-based settings.

These systemic factors are almost certainly a major reason for the higher rates of hospital use in Australia. An additional systemic factor is the absence of US-style managed care organisations that have a real ability to minimise use of expensive hospital facilities by ensuring patients receive alternative specialist care as outpatients in lower-cost, community-based facilities. The evidence from the US experience with managed care indicates that major savings are more likely to be made on the cost of hospital care by managing hospital ultilisation. This suggests that it is unwise for advocates of health reform to place all their eggs in the primary care/chronic disease management basket.

A Value-Based National Health Innovation Agenda

In contemporary Australia, the chief economic reform challenge is to curb the ever-rising cost of health to government budgets. Hence, the Turnbull government has been encouraged by the Harper Competition Review to extend the market-based reform principles of the 1980s to the task of health reform. This would entail greater application of the principles of consumer choice, fostering greater competition between providers, encouraging the entry of private competitors into the health economy, and separation of regulatory, funding, and service delivery roles.[88] These are worthy goals, which have been optimistically taken up by advocates of the government's primary care reform agenda as establishing the framework within which these reforms will occur as a means of "opening up the health system to more contestability."[89]

Economic reform was in the 1980s known as structural or micro-economic reform, and consisted of measures that sought to boost local productivity and increase international competitiveness. One phase of that era of reform involved the deregulation of statutory monopolies through the privatisation of government agencies in areas such as electricity, ports, and other infrastructure such as roads and transport. Significantly, for political reasons Medicare has been largely quarantined from this agenda—and continues to be quarantined despite the mounting evidence that the system is out-dated and inefficient.

Overseas experience has shown that health reform initiatives must aim to bridge the institutional divide between non-hospital and hospital-based health services, which exist due to traditional fee-for-service payment systems that reward providers for inefficient practice and encourage over-serving. To reiterate: the insights gained from the American experience with 'bundled' payments and integrated care to address spiralling US healthcare costs suggest that major savings are most likely to be made on the cost of hospital care by managing utilisation. The ACQ experiment has bent the cost curve down and yielded cost-effective savings by reducing use of procedures, images and tests, and by directing patients away from high-cost hospitals towards alternative, lower-cost, community-based facilities for specialist procedures. Likewise, Kaiser Permanente has limited health costs primarily by rigorous management of hospital admissions and length of stays rather than by chronic disease management. This is especially significant to the health reform debate in this country, given very high rates of hospital use in Australia compared to other OECD nations—including the US and UK—and given that the rising cost of health to government budgets is being largely driven by the increasing cost of hospital care.

The reality, therefore, is that persisting with the Medicare status quo, and pouring additional taxpayer funding into the public health services to pay for coordinated care under the banner of so-called primary care reform, would represent the antithesis of genuine structural reform and health innovation. The further implication is that the calls by the Premiers of NSW and South Australia to increase the GST, along with all other mooted tax hikes to pay for the rising cost of public hospital care to state and territory government budgets, could well serve to prop up latently inefficient hospital-based health services, and represents the antithesis of economic reform. An economically rational approach to modernising the health system could free up and redeploy health resources in a more optimal and sustainable fashion to meet the healthcare needs of the nation.

In its recent review of the efficiency of the health system, the Productivity Commission argued there was some scope to achieve greater efficiencies that would improve the quality of, and access to, publicly-funded healthcare by undertaking 'within system' reforms that did not alter the current structure of Medicare.[90] But the Commission also argued that "the system's institutional and funding structures compromise its performance" and that "larger-scale reforms may be required to make real and enduring inroads into allocative and dynamic efficiency." In this context, the Commission singled out the need for reforms that addressed dominance of fee-for-service payments for both primary and hospital care, and flagged new integrated payment models that better aligned financial incentives and health outcomes. It also indicated the potential for private health insurers to play a leading role in addressing the systemic problems of complexity, perverse incentives, fragmentation and lack of coordination. Recognising the scale of the changes contemplated, it suggested that private health regulations barring health funds from involvement in primary care be relaxed in order to trial innovative integrated care initiatives that would help build the evidence base for reform. It also recommended that the process of long-term reform be "informed by a comprehensive and independent review of the health system."[91]

Such a review undertaken by a body like the Productivity Commission might well provide the intellectual ammunition required to build the case for structural health reform. But it cannot provide the political will and political capital, which can only be generated by committing to a policy rather than a process. Another review, moreover, would simply repeat the extensive work of the NHHRC, which has already concluded that a Netherlands-style voucher model was the best option for systemic reform to achieve efficiencies and innovation through consumer choice and provider competition.[92]

Private Sector Managed Care—Medicare Select

Private health insurers in Australia face similar policy challenges to the public health system. They too confront the problem of a relatively small number of members who suffer complex chronic illness generating the bulk of health service costs, including frequent admissions to hospitals. The insurers also face the problem of adverse selection and individuals— particularly as they age—taking out, maintaining and upgrading their private cover when they believe their health status means they are most likely to access healthcare. Community rating rules mean health funds are obliged to insure all comers and are not allowed to refuse cover or charge higher premiums to 'bad risk' elderly or chronically ill patients.

2. Integrated Care and Alternative Payment Models

In relation to addressing the issues that push up premium and benefit costs, and threaten to make private cover unaffordable, insurers' hands are also tied on two further fronts in trying to manage the financial risks involved in covering the cost of members' healthcare. Federal health insurance regulations prevent private health funds from covering any out-of-hospital services already funded through Medicare. This includes paying for the kind of community-based GP and other medical services that might, under the right conditions, reduce hospital admissions. Health funds also have limited ability to manage the utilisation of hospital services because they are subject to a strict insurance indemnity, which mandates that funds must pay for member's hospital care if the admission is approved by a registered medical practitioner—an arrangement that inherently carries the risk of supplier-induced demand and over-servicing, especially for procedural surgical care. These regulations are currently under reconsideration as part of yet another federal government review: the Private Health Insurance Consultations.[93]

The common problems faced across the public and private systems suggest that the resources deployed in both systems could be better used if combined to address the same challenges. This is part of the logic behind the national health reform plan, under which it has been suggested the existing Medicare scheme be replaced with a new publicly-funded, privately-operated health insurance scheme called Medicare Select, to create a more dynamic health economy.

The proposal is that all Australians would receive taxpayer-funded health insurance vouchers, with the value of the voucher being risk-adjusted for factors such as age, gender, health status, and socio-economic criteria. Vouchers would be used to partly pay for the cost of purchasing insurance from a competing range of health and hospital plans that would cover a minimum mandatory set of essential services. Health funds would be responsible for purchasing services from hospitals and other providers on behalf of their members.

The advantages of Medicare Select compared to the status quo would include greater consumer choice and provider competition. In the new competitive environment, publicly-funded health cover would be portable and funds would compete on price and quality to win and retain members. To enhance competition on the insurance side of the new system, funds would also charge private premiums paid for out of individual's own pockets, with additional government top-up subsidies for low income groups. The key changes would, however, be on the services side of the health system. Instead of operating as passive payers of medical and hospital bills, health funds would operate as active purchasers of healthcare from competing producers. To limit premium and benefit costs, and attract and retain members, funds would seek to ensure the services they purchase are provided at the best price and highest quality, and successful providers will have to meet these cost and quality criteria to win service contracts.

After extensively reviewing and cataloguing the problems with the current health system, the NHHRC final report endorsed the Medicare Select model as its preferred long-term health reform option.[94] One of the chief recommendations for a Medicare Select-style, risk-rated, private sector 'managed care' scheme is that it would remedy the structural defects that plague Medicare, and account for chronic care gaps and overuse of hospitals. Private health funds would hold the full financial risk for members' healthcare needs across the full service spectrum. They would thus have a superior incentive to ensure health resources are used as efficiently as possible so patients receive the most appropriate and cost-effective care—including all beneficial primary care and outpatient specialist care to avoid expensive hospital admissions. This would include seeking to reduce the cost of insuring chronically-ill members by ensuring their conditions are properly managed by appropriate primary care to prevent expensive episodes of acute illness requiring hospitalisation. Enabling health funds to operate active purchasing agents would establish the kind of contestable market environment that would spur providers to innovate and discover the most cost-effective means of delivering health services.

Under these conditions, a substantial reorganisation of health service provision could be envisaged. Chronic care could well be offered by disease-specific specialised clinics that will emerge to fill a clear gap in the market. Funds would negotiate contracts with these clinics, which would be the default 'medical homes' of members, and would be paid not solely for delivering 'inputs'—on a fee-for-service basis—but based on their ability to deliver innovative and high-quality 'outputs' in the form of cost-effective packages of care providing ongoing courses of treatment that maintain and improve the health of patients. As importantly, American experience with private sector managed care suggests there is considerable scope to directly address the over-use of hospitals in traditional health systems by delivering care in alternative lower-cost settings, either in specialists' outpatient rooms or in fit-for-purpose community-based specialist clinics. This is particularly important if, as the evidence suggests, improving the quality of primary care uncovers unmet need for hospital care, which better managed care could divert for treatment into lowest cost settings. This is to say that the Medicare Select option possibly offers a pathway to alternative payment models that are cost-effective.

A 'Big Bang' Too Far

Introducing a purchaser-provider split into the public system, particularly to enable the private provision of public hospital services,[95] is a natural extension of the reform principles of the 1980s. Yet the reform challenge is immense because these principles are foreign to the culture and political economy of the public system, and run up against myriad institutional and political obstacles—including public sector union opposition, to say nothing of the entrenched opposition of the organised medical profession to any proposal that even hints at the principle and practice of managed care. Institutional factors also include the lack of sophisticated contracting skills in public health bureaucracies. The later factor strongly suggests the tendency under any public sector chronic/managed care regime will likely be to default to the standard approach of top-down bureaucratic, primary-care focused program funding—which copious evidence indicates is a dead end if the intention is to develop genuinely innovative, effective and efficient, new and fully integrated, models of healthcare.

A different approach, consistent with the principles of economic reform, would be to bypass the bureaucracy in favour of outsourcing the task to the private sector more familiar with striking competitive commercial relationships between purchasers and providers. This is to recommend the Medicare Select model, and to envisage a situation wherein health funds managed the healthcare needs and financial risk of their membership by purchasing the most appropriate, effective and efficient services from financially-accountable and risk-sharing health providers. A fair question is whether health funds currently possess the skills to act as informed purchasers, given the long history of private health insurance essentially operating as a payment system guaranteeing that doctors' bills will be paid. The reform challenge for the private health industry is to accept that genuine reform would require a commitment to change long-established corporate mindsets and institutional structures to prepare for a new era of financial risk management and cost-effective management of care.

The challenge for government is to recognise that a starting point for true economic reform and innovation in the health system would be to create a situation on the demand-side of the health economy where there are cost- and quality-conscious purchasers, which in turn would stimulate innovations on the supply-side of the health economy to deliver the best quality and best value care. In this respect, it is worth noting the Medicare Select model is not as radical as it may sound: one of its first proponents was the health economist Richard Scotton, who was one of the architects of the original Medicare scheme in the 1960s. Scotton still believed in the provision of public subsidies to ensure access to essential health services regardless of means; the question he was prepared to face honestly was whether there were more efficient and effective ways of delivering those subsidies, and the care needed, than a 'free', universal, taxpayer-funded, fee-for-service payment system.[96]

It is also worth emphasising that the debate about alternative health payment models is anything but new. It dates to well before Scotton's disenchantment with Medicare, and back at least to the medical profession's success in breaking up the 'Friendly Societies' contract payment system in the 1950s at the time when federal government fee-for-service benefits for medical services were first made available under the Menzies government's National Health Scheme.[97] Discussion of alternative models has, however, always been shut down politically due to the strident and vocal opposition of the medical profession to any proposal to tamper with the fundamentals of the current fee-for-service arrangements.[98]

The political obstacles to 'big bang' system-wide health reform as envisaged under Medicare Select are thus formidable. The AMA has long signalled its preparedness to undertake 'managed scare' campaigns at any mention of introducing managed care regimes in Australia, in defence of the medical professions vested interest in the retention of the 'sacred (cash) cow' that is the fee-for-service Medicare system which principally benefits GPs and specialists by underwriting their private medical businesses.

Despite the intransigence of self-interested providers, structural changes to the health system—going well beyond limited primary healthcare 'reforms'—are necessary to transform the way health services are purchased and provided, to deliver to the community the best value healthcare for its increasingly scarce health dollars. The first challenge, however, is to find a politically-feasible way of implementing the alternative payment and service models that could potentially reduce the cost of health by effectively and efficiently controlling use of hospital services. A politically-viable health reform strategy that avoids the pitfalls of big bang proposals and can deliver meaningful change in the health sector is the subject of the next chapter discussing Health Innovation Communities.

Endnotes

1   'Health reforms could save hospitals $1.5 bn', The Australian, 9 December, 2015.
2   John Dwyer, 'Private health insurance reform: prevention the key to cure', The Australian, 27 November, 2015.
3   Australian Institute of Health and Welfare, Australia's Health 2014, Canberra: AIHW 2014, p.54.
4   I am grateful to a reviewer who helped to clarify these points.

5   Peter Phelan and Jeremy Sammut, Overcoming Cost and Governance Challenges for Australian Public Hospitals: The Foundation Trust Alternative, Policy Monograph 137, (Sydney: The Centre for Independent Studies 2013), 6.

6   Australian Government, Reform of the Federation White Paper, 32.

7   FM Harris, Jayasinghe UW, Taggart JR et al. 'Multidisciplinary Team Care Arrangements in the management of patients with chronic disease in Australian general practice', Medical Journal of Australia, 2011; 194: 236–239; Zwar NA, Hermiz O, Comino EJ, et al. 'Do multidisciplinary care plans result in better care for type 2 diabetes?' Aust Fam Physician 2007; 36: 85-89.

8   Simon Cowan (ed.), Emergency Budget Repair Kit (Sydney: The Centre for Independent Studies, 2014.

9   Medicare Benefits Schedule Review Taskforce, Public Submissions Consultation Paper, September 2015, 1.

10 Medicare Benefits Schedule Review Taskforce, Public Submissions Consultation Paper, 15.

11 Primary Health Care Advisory Group, Better Outcomes for People with Chronic and Complex Health Conditions through Primary Health Care Discussion Paper, August 2015, 4.

12 'Federal budget 2014: Commonwealth to slash share of hospital funding', Sydney Morning Herald, 13 May, 2013.

13 'States taxing powers a fundamental federation reform, Turnbull says,' The Australian, 30 March, 2016.

14 COAG Meeting Communique, 1 April 2016. http://www.coag.gov.au/node/537#1

15 'One-stop shop for chronic care unveiled by government,' The Australian, 31 March, 2016.

16 Jeremy Sammut, Like the Curate's Egg: A Market-based Response and Alternative to the Bennett Report, Policy Monograph 104, (Sydney: The Centre for Independent Studies, 2009).

17 Primary Health Care Advisory Group, Better Outcomes for People with Chronic and Complex Health Conditions through Primary Health Care Discussion Paper, 5, 8-9.

18 Sammut, Curate's Egg, vii.

19 Primary Health Care Advisory Group, Better Outcomes for People with Chronic and Complex Health Conditions through Primary Health Care Discussion Paper, 15-6.

20 National Health and Hospital Reform Commission (NHHRC), A Healthier Future for all Australians: Final Report, June 2009 (Commonwealth of Australia, Canberra, 2009) (Final Report), 7, 9, 84, 95, 136.

21 Primary Health Care Advisory Group Final Report Better Outcomes for People with Chronic and Complex Health Conditions, Report to the Government on the Findings of Primary Health Care Advisory Group, December 2016.

22 Minister For Health Minister For Aged Care Minister For Sport The Hon. Sussan Ley MP A Healthier Medicare for chronically-ill patients, , Joint Media Release 31 March 2016.

23 NHHRC, Final Report, 10, 23.

24 This section draws on the findings of Jeremy Sammut, The False Promise of GP Super Clinics Part 2: Coordinated Care CIS Policy Monograph No. 85 Papers in Health and Ageing (4) (Sydney: The Centre for Independent Studies, 2008).

25 Commonwealth Department of Health and Aged Care, The Australian Coordinated Care Trials: Summary of the Final Technical National Evaluation Report on the First Round of Trials (Canberra: Commonwealth of Australia, 2002).

26 Commonwealth Department of Health and Ageing, The National Evaluation of the Second Round of Coordinated Care Trials (Canberra: Commonwealth of Australia, 2007), 595, 621–622, 627, 630–631.

27 Malcolm W. Battersby, 'Health Reform through Coordinated Care: SA Health Plus,' British Medical Journal 330:7492 (19 March 2005), 662–665.

28 Adrian J. Esterman and David I. Ben-Tovim, 'The Australian Coordinated Care Trials: Success
or Failure?,' Medical Journal of Australia 177 (4 November 2002), 470.

29 Sammut, The False Promise of GP Super Clinics Part 2.

30 Esterman and Ben-Tovim, 'The Australian Coordinated Care Trials'

31 Paul Cunningham and Jeremy Sammut, 'Inadequate acute hospital beds and the limits of primary care and prevention', Emergency Medicine Australia, (2012) 24, 566-572.

32 Leonie Segal, A Vision for Primary Care: Funding and other System Factors for Optimising the Primary Care Contribution to the Community's Health (August 2008), 2.

33 Lyle Nelson, "Care Coordination, and Value-Based Payment", Issue Brief, Health and Human Resources, Congressional Budget Office, January 2012.

34 John C. Goodman, Priceless: Curing the Healthcare Crisis, (The Independent Institute: Oakland, 2012), 72-74

35 H. Gravelle and others, 'Impact of Case Management (Evercare) on Frail Elderly Patients: Controlled Before and After Analysis of Quantitative Outcome Data,' British Medical Journal 334:7583 (6 January 2007), 31–34. The evaluation confirmed the findings of two earlier reviews that 'showed no consistent evidence for the effectiveness of case management in preventing hospital attendances or admissions, reducing health costs, or improving function.' David Oliver, 'Government Should Have Respected Evidence,' British Medical Journal 334:7585 (20 January 2007), 109.

36 The University of Auckland, 'Evaluation of Care Plus Programme, New Zealand' Health Policy Monitor Survey (9) (2007). For a full evaluation, see CBG Health Research, Review of the Implementation of Care Plus (Wellington: New Zealand Ministry of Health, 2006), 2.

37 Hal Swerissen and Stephen Duckett, Chronic Failure in Primary Care, Grattan Institute Report No. 2016-2, March 2016.

38 Goodman, Priceless, 73-4.

39 S. de Bruin, C. A Baan, and J. N. Struijs, 'Pay-for performance in disease management: a systematic review of the literature', BMC Health Service Research, 2011, 11:272

40 Flodgren, G., Eccles, M.P., Shepperd, S., Scott, A., Parmelli, E. and Beyer, F.R. 2011, 'An overview of reviews evaluating the effectiveness of financial incentives in changing healthcare professional behaviours and patient outcomes', Cochrane Database of Systematic Reviews, no. 7; A. Scott, Sivey, P., Ait Ouakrim, D., Willenberg, L., Naccarella, L., Furler, J. and Young, D. 2011, 'The effect of financial incentives on the quality of healthcare provided by primary care physicians', Cochrane Database of Systematic Reviews, no. 9.

41 See Megan McArdle, "Why Pilot Projects Fail", The Atlantic, December 21, 2011.

42 National Primary Care Research and Development Centre, 'National Evaluation of Expert Patients Programme: Key Findings (Research into Expert Patients—Outcomes in a Randomised Trial,' Executive Summary 44 (March 2007.

43 Marshall, L., Charlesworth, A. and Hurst, J. 2014, The NHS Payment System: Evolving Policy and Emerging Evidence, Nuffield Trust, London, 11.

44 Marshall, L., Charlesworth, A. and Hurst, J. 2014, The NHS Payment System, 15.

45 Marshall, L., Charlesworth, A. and Hurst, J. 2014, The NHS Payment System, 24-5.

46 Marshall, L., Charlesworth, A. and Hurst, J. 2014, The NHS Payment System, 15, 24; See also Productivity Commission, Research Paper, (Canberra: 2015), 29-30.

47 Marshall, L., Charlesworth, A. and Hurst, J. 2014, The NHS Payment System, 15, 24; See also Productivity Commission, Efficiency in Health, 11, 25.

48 Primary Health Care Advisory Group Final Report; Minister For Health Minister For Aged Care Minister For Sport The Hon. Sussan Ley MP A Healthier Medicare for chronically-ill patients.

49 A. Podger, 'A Model Health System for Australia', public presentation given for the Menzies Centre
for Health Policy, 3 March 2006.

50 Ged Kearney, 'Nurses perfectly able to do more', The Australian. 14 February 2009.

51 Goodman, Priceless, 7-9.

52 Porter, M.E. and Lee, T.H. 2013, 'The strategy that will fix health care', Harvard Business Review, October, pp. 50–70.

53 Marshall, L., Charlesworth, A. and Hurst, J. 2014, The NHS Payment System, 15, 24; See also Productivity Commission, Efficiency in Health, Research Paper, (Canberra: 2015), 4, 25.

54 A. Charlesworth, L. Hawkins and L. Marshall, NHS Payment Reform: Lessons from the Past and Directions for the Future, Nuffield Trust, London, 2014, 3.

55 E. Fisher, et.al, Health Care Spending, Quality, and Outcomes: More Isn't Always Better, Dartmouth Institute, 2009, 4.

56 Productivity Commission, Efficiency in Health, 36.

57 Hildebrandt, H., Schulte, T. and Stunder, B. 2012, 'Triple Aim in Kinzigtal, Germany: Improving population health, integrating health care and reducing costs of care—Lessons for the UK?', Journal of Integrated Care, vol. 20, no. 4, pp. 205–222.

58 James Bartholomew, The Welfare of Nations, Biteback Publishing: London, 2015,

59 Business Council of Australia, The Future of Health: A Discussion Starter, October 2015, 6.

60 Charlesworth, A., Davies, A. and Dixon, J. 2012, Reforming Payment for Health Care in Europe to Achieve Better Value, Nuffield Trust, London, 6-7.

61 Business Council of Australia, The Future of Health: A Discussion Starter, October 2015, 25.

62 Charlesworth, A., Davies, A. and Dixon, J. 2012, Reforming Payment for Health Care in Europe to Achieve Better Value, 30-34.

63 Bartholomew, The Welfare of Nations,

64 D.H. de Bakker, et.al, 'Early Results from Adoption of Bundled Payments for Diabetes Care In The Netherlands Show Improvement in Care Coordination', Health Affairs, 31, 2, 2012, 426-433.

65 Charlesworth, A., Davies, A. and Dixon, J. 2012, Reforming Payment for Health Care in Europe to Achieve Better Value, 4, 13, 26, 33.

66 This section draws on findings of Jeremy Sammut, The False Promise of GP Super Clinics Part 2.

67 R. G. A. Feachem and others, 'Getting More for their Dollar: A Comparison of the NHS with California's Kaiser Permanente,' British Medical Journal 324:7330 (19 January 2002), 135.

68 N. Zwar and others, A Systematic Review of Chronic Disease Management, 13; King's Fund, Managing Chronic Disease: What Can We Learn From the US Experience?, (London: King's Fund Publications, 2004).

69 R. G. A. Feachem and others, 'Getting More for Their Dollar,' 139

70 B. Firemen and others, 'Can Disease Management Reduce Health Care Costs by Improving Quality?'

71 R. G. A. Feachem and others, 'Getting More for Their Dollar,' 138, 140.

72 As above, 140.

73 Productivity Commission, Efficiency in Health, 36.

74 R.E. Mechanic, et.al, 'Medical Group Responses To Global Payment: Early Lessons from the "Alternative Quality Contract" in Massachusetts', Health Affairs, 30, 9, 2011, 17341742, 1734-5.

75 Z. Song, et.al, "Changes in Health Care Spending and Quality 4 Years into Global Payment', New England Journal of Medicine, 371, 18, 2014, 1704-1714,1705

76 R.E. Mechanic, et.al, 'Medical Group Responses To Global Payment', 1737.

77 Song, et.al, "Changes in Health Care Spending and Quality 4 Years into Global Payment', 1705

78 R.E. Mechanic, et.al, 'Medical Group Responses To Global Payment', 1738.

79 R.E. Mechanic, et.al, 'Medical Group Responses To Global Payment', 1738-9.

80 R.E. Mechanic, et.al, 'Medical Group Responses To Global Payment' 1739.

81 R.E. Mechanic, et.al, 'Medical Group Responses To Global Payment', 1737-8.

82 R.E. Mechanic, et.al, 'Medical Group Responses To Global Payment', 1737-8

83 Song, et.al, "Changes in Health Care Spending and Quality 4 Years into Global Payment',1708-12

84 John Daley and Cassie McGannon, Budget pressures on Australian governments, 2014 edition, Grattan Institute.

85 Angus Taylor, 'Tax Hikes are not Tax Reforms', Australian Polity, vol. 5, no. 4. 2015, 18-19.

86 Gadiel and Sammut, Lessons from Singapore: Opt-Out Health Savings Accounts for Australia, Policy Monograph 140, (Sydney: The Centre for Independent Studies, 2014)13.

87 Business Council of Australia, Overview of Megatrends in Health and their Implications for Australia, Background Paper, October 2015, 5.

88 Harper, I. et al., Competition Policy Review, Final Report, (Canberra: Commonwealth of Australia, 2015).

89 Taylor, 19.

90 Productivity Commission, Efficiency in Health, 1.

91 Productivity Commission, Efficiency in Health, 4, 30, 39, 67, 94-5.

92 NHHRC, Final Report, 147.

93 Australian Department of Health, Issues for Consideration at roundtables on private health insurance, November 2015.

94 Final Report, 147.

95 David Gadiel and Jeremy Sammut, How the NSW Coalition Should Govern Health: Strategies for Microeconomic Reform, Policy Monograph 128 (Sydney: The Centre for Independent Studies 2012).

96 Productivity Commission, Managed Competition in health care. Workshop Proceeding. (Canberra: 2002).

97 Jeremy Sammut, How! Not How Much: Medicare Spending and Health Resource Allocation in Australia, Policy Monograph 114 (Sydney: The Centre for Independent Studies, 2011).

98 Sidney Sax, A Strife of Interests: Politics and Policies in Australian Health Services (Sydney: George Allen & Unwin, 1984.

Chapter 3

Health Innovation Communities*

Jeremy Sammut, Peta Seaton, & Gerald Thomas

The Trouble with Health Reform

The allocative and technical inefficiencies in Australia's $161 billion health system mean that many Australians are not receiving the right care in the right place at the best price possible. Conservative estimates suggest these inefficiencies currently cost the nation at least $17.7 billion a year. (Figure 2). Although the 11% of the total national health spend that is wasted represents a significant net welfare loss that could potentially be saved, redeployed or redirected, lack of reform at the systemic level prevents service redesigns that could deliver better value for money and more cost-effective healthcare for Australians.[1]

The trouble with health reform in Australia is *not* that we do not know the kind of structural problems that need to be addressed to create a more sustainable health system in Australia. There is a range of policy options that would deliver better value for money and more cost-effective healthcare. Many of these reform ideas have been canvassed in recent major reports both by official government bodies and health industry groups. Many of these solutions are well known, having long been discussed in health policy circles and featuring in a litany of reports, reviews, and inquiries into the health system over many years.

---

* First published as Medi-Vation: Health Innovation Communities for Medicare Payment and Service Reform Research Report 21, (Sydney: The Centre for Independent Studies, 2016).

Figure 2: Traditional Health Spending & Intergrated Health Spending†, Australia 2004-2015

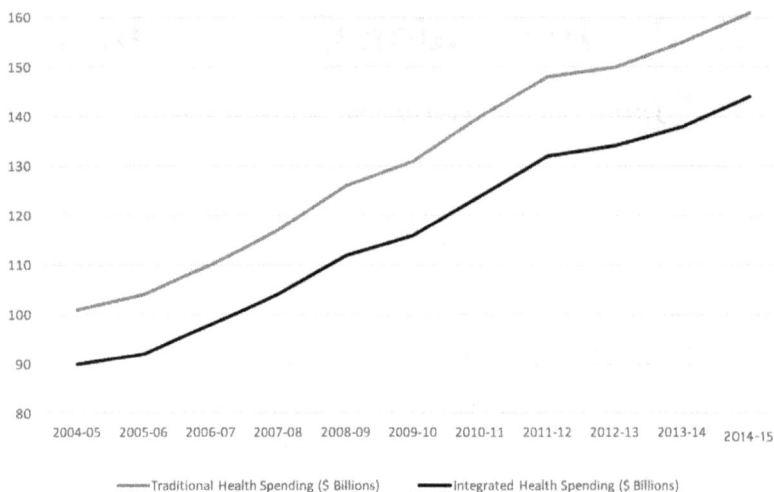

For example, the 2015 OECD review of the Australian health system flagged, yet again, the perennial problems posed by the fragmented nature of the system. The fact that in both the public and private systems, no single funder is responsible for the entire healthcare needs of patients, skews incentives, reduces efficiency, and increases costs by preventing the integration and coordination of primary and hospital care.[2]

But despite the great deal of attention paid to expounding these well-known problems, the vital element lacking in the health debate is an effective, politically-feasible reform strategy that will allow the solutions to be implemented to improve the outcomes and performance of the health system. Because the political obstacles to achieving significant change and redesigns of health funding and service arrangements are so formidable, much of what passes as the discussion of the future of the health system seems to be obsessed with simply describing the problems. The debate needs to instead focus on developing practical and achievable solutions

---

† Based on 11% efficiency gap estimated in Health Reform: Higher Quality, Lower Costs. A Port Jackson Partners Limited Report to Private Healthcare Australia, May 2014.

to overcome the technical and institutional impediments to change that plague the health sector.

Review of the existing health debate therefore serves the dual purpose of not only clarifying the problems within the existing health system, but of identifying the limitations of the debate itself with regard to initiatives and mechanisms that can lead to genuine innovation within the sector. This chapter argues that these deficiencies — both the structural problems and the shortcomings of the so-called 'solutions' that are offered — can be overcome by taking the national discussion of health reform in a new direction. A national health innovation policy that establishes the 'Health Innovation Communities' proposed and described herein, is the first step towards reaching the long sought-after solution for the healthcare funding and delivery problems that continue to stubbornly resist change.

Public Sector Rigidities

Another good, recent example of the trouble with the health reform debate is the April 2015 Productivity Commission Research Paper, *Efficiency in Health*, which re-identified three "well-understood" structural inefficiencies within the Australian health system.

The first inefficiency identified by the Productivity Commission is inadequate focus on preventive health to address problems — such as obesity — that are a leading cause of chronic disease. The second inefficiency is inadequate focus on the ongoing management of chronic disease in a community or non-hospital based primary care setting. The combined effect of the first and second defect contributes to the third defect, which is the significant number of high-cost hospital admissions (up to an estimated 10% of total admissions) that were potentially avoidable had prior, appropriate and lower-cost preventive and chronic care been available.[3] This is in keeping with the 'hospital-centric' character of the Australian health system, with its considerably higher rates of hospital use compared to comparable OECD countries, which is due to systemic factors, especially 'fee for service' payments for specialist services.[4]

The Productivity Commission rightly argued that these structural inefficiencies are allocative in nature. Alternative models of care that would spend existing health dollars more effectively are not adequately resourced as a result of the "effects of current institutional and funding structures on the performance of Australia's health system."[5] Policy objectives and financial incentives are misaligned because, in both the public and private health systems, the bulk of health funding is locked up in inflexible fee-for-service payment models. Healthcare providers, mainly doctors, are principally rewarded on a basis of providing one-off episodes of either medical (mainly GP) care or hospital care when acute illness or disease strikes.[6] Rather than a comprehensive health insurance and risk management system, the rigid public health system and regimented private insurance system both primarily function as provider-captured payment mechanisms for separate sets of hospital-based care and community-based primary care.[7]

Fee-for-service payments not only prohibit the development of alternative models of integrated healthcare covering the full service spectrum and full cycle of care; they also encourage doctors to increase activity to maximize income, and thus lead to costly and unnecessary over-servicing—including elevated rates of hospital use.[8] As explained in the previous chapter, jurisdictional complexity also accounts for the fragmented nature of health service provision. Under Australia's complex division of health responsibilities, the federal government is primarily responsible for healthcare delivered outside hospitals, and state governments responsible for public hospital care. No single level of government or funder has full responsibility for all the health care needs of patients, and no direct control over the kind of services patients receive and the locations where those services are provided.[9]

Lack of systemic reform to remove structural rigidities is throttling service delivery innovation that could improve the quality of care, save scarce health resources, and redeploy existing funding more efficiently. With regards to public hospitals, for example, joint federal-state funding is paid on 'activity-basis' at the so-called efficient price determined by the average cost of particular hospital services across the system. Activity funding (which is essentially another form of fee-for-service) not only continues to encourage over-servicing; it also rigidly ties funding to existing hospital-based models of care—at a large recurrent and capital cost to the public finances—and prevents service redesigns that may increase efficiency and improve outcomes.[10]

Private Health Regimentation

Complexity, fragmentation and inflexibility also apply in relation to privately-funded health services, due to the regulations that apply to private health insurance. The strict indemnity covering private insurers mandates that health funds must pay for member's hospital care if the admission is approved by a registered medical practitioner. The indemnity—and hence the blunting of price signals for insured services—has major implications for usage of hospital services, especially of discretionary procedural care and when copayments are completely avoided via 'No Gap' cover.[11] These demand-side problems on the private insurance market are compounded by the problems on the supply side: the *Health Insurance Act* also bans health funds from paying benefits for any out-of-hospital medical service for which Medicare rebates are available. The rationale for these regulations is to prevent a two-tiered health system, in which privately insured patients secure preferential access to doctor's services due to the higher payments available. These concerns are debatable given the experience in other comparable health systems: private insurers in New Zealand are free to cover the full spectrum of healthcare costs without undermining 'free and universal' objectives of the government-run health system, and without raising even the fear—let alone the reality—of a two-tiered system.[12]

In Australia, however, the restrictions on private cover prevent private health insurers from funding preventive and chronic services and developing alternative cost-effective models of care that may reduce the disease burden, manage chronic illness more effectively, and minimise expensive hospitalisations. In practice, private health insurers are able to push the cost of the more complex task of managing the community-based treatment of their customers on to the public system—which is where most fund members with chronic disease receive primary care—leaving the private system with the simpler, principle task of providing hospital-based procedural services.[13]

In both the public and private systems, therefore, providers are paid for doing the same things in the same way as mandated by current funding and payment systems, which means consumers get access to only the kind and mix of services that funders/payers agree to fund/pay for. The MBS Schedule, for example, proscribes the way patients can and can't be treated by only paying for certain 'items' of care on a fee-for-service basis. Public hospitals —as with private health funds— are also prohibited from reorganising their services and providing care outside hospitals, even if it is cost-effective and clinically appropriate. This is despite international evidence (discussed in Chapter 2) showing health systems that break down the traditional divide between hospital and non-hospital care are more efficient. The existing service systems also provide no incentive and limited assistance for individuals to take responsibility for their own avoidable health risks. Input-focused and transactional in nature, providers are rewarded simply for delivering discrete health interventions irrespective of the results, rather than being rewarded based on 'outputs'— overall improvements in health status and wellbeing.[14]

With specific regards to the private health system, community rating regulations—which prohibit the charging of different premiums based on health risk—also permit health funds to shift the cost of high risk patients ('high-cost' claims and customers aged over 55) on to a secondary re-insurance risk pool. The Reinsurance Trust Fund currently administered by the Private Health Insurance Administration Council compensates those funds paying higher than average benefits by redistributing money contributed from funds paying less than average benefits. The effect is to blunt incentives for funds to develop new products and services to manage health risks and costs, since funds that bear the cost of additional preventive or chronic care will not receive a full return on any savings generated—which are instead shared across the industry.[15] Hence one of the few risk-management and cost-containment strategies available to health funds is the relatively blunt instrument of re-negotiating the value of benefits paid to hospitals and specialists, in addition to pioneering efforts by some funds to 'pay for quality' by refusing to pay benefits for additional care occasioned by avoidable adverse events and preventable errors.[16]

As the consulting firm Port Jackson Partners argued in a 2014 report for private health fund peak body Private Healthcare Australia, embracing more cost-effective integrated care requires following the lead of international leaders in healthcare reform and taking steps to remove the artificial barriers between primary care and hospital care that plague the Australian health system. This would include removing current regulations that restrict private health funds' involvement in primary care. Necessary reforms would also include exploring alternative capitation-based payment models that covered the full spectrum of both primary and hospital care, and which would allow greater involvement of private sector health management companies in the organisation and coordination of care pathways. The report argued that integrated payments would also remove the incentives to over-service on hospital care created by fee-for-service payments, and encourage the development of new ways of delivering the same care in lower-cost settings, such as in community-based clinics, or through the provision of sub-acute care in a 'hotel-style' accommodation, as occurs in more efficient health systems overseas.[17]

The Limitations of Current Reform Strategies

'Within System'?

The Productivity Commission has drawn a useful distinction between what it has called 'within system' reforms—which could deliver beneficial outcomes without "changing existing institutional and funding structures"—and larger scale reforms of the existing architecture of the health system that would involve enormous dislocations of current practice, carry the risk of unintended consequences regardless of the expertise and experience informing the design, and be stymied by political obstacles including the vocal opposition from vested interests wedded to the status quo.[18]

In a December 2015 submission to the Turnbull government's review of private health insurance, Private Healthcare Australia identified a list of what were called "near-term priorities for change." Notably absent from this list was demanding the federal government take action to open the primary care sector up to private health funds. Instead, the submission was content with merely warning that the incremental changes were "not a substitute for the broader reform necessary for the Australian healthcare system to deliver much higher quality outcomes at lower cost."[19]

Similarly, the submission by Australia's largest private health fund, Medibank Private, argued—with respect to ever-rising use and cost of insured health services and the flow-on impact on the affordability of private insurance premiums—that "today's regulatory settings have lost relevance and weakened competition leading to low-value practices that come at the expense of consumers." It was strongly asserted that "insurers should have the incentive and mandate to better manage their aged and chronically ill populations outside of hospital." But action in this direction was also absent from its list of "near-term recommendations on which government should act"—though the submission did flag support for "potentially moving towards a value-based or capitated model."[20]

Big Bang/Damp Squib

The problem, of course, is that 'within system' reforms will leave the major structural problems and inefficiencies that compromise the system's performance untouched. The Port Jackson Partners/Private Healthcare Australia report argued that potentially large and significant quality and cost gains:

> ...are not possible within the current healthcare framework—they demand more significant structural reforms, and the introduction of competition, such has been driven in most other sectors of the Australian economy.[21]

This call for structural reform went beyond permitting private insurers to get involved in primary care, and included a call to 'privatise' Medicare by contracting out a 'Universal Service Obligation' to private health funds that would manage and purchase the care of their members—a market-based Medicare Select-style framework that would facilitate the entry into the health sector of innovative private sector providers of integrated, better quality, and lower cost care.[22]

The problem, however, is that proposals for 'big bang' changes to the health system may ultimately prove to be a damp squib. Despite the well-known fiscal imperative to control the escalating cost of health and achieve better value for money, fundamental reforms are highly likely to be blocked by institutional and cultural factors—especially the competing interest of rival stakeholders, together with the Australian electorate's well-demonstrated conservatism regarding significant changes to the operation of Medicare.

With respect to reform of private health, the Productivity Commission has commented that changes to the private health insurance regulations, while justifiable by the potential benefits, could undermine the equity objectives of Medicare if resulting in a two-tiered level of access to care. The Productivity Commission also flagged the likely opposition of the organised medical profession. The influential doctors' lobby group, the Australian Medical Association (AMA) has long been virulently opposed to private funds having a greater involvement in the organisation and coordination of primary care, and opposed to any suggestion of new models of 'managed care' that could restrict doctors' access to fee-for-service payments. Given the considerable obstacles to fundamental change, what the Productivity Commission has therefore proposed is an "incremental approach to reform"—a trial and test process. It has suggested that the federal government could permit health funds to operate designated preventive or chronic care services in particular regions or for a particular patient group, which would be evaluated to assess all the benefits, costs, and potential adverse consequence to build the case for reform.[23]

Trials and Tribulations

There are obvious advantages to the process proposed by the Productivity Commission in order to circumvent the difficulties associated with large-scale reforms that would struggle to win support and be implemented. However, the beneficial outcomes achieved by the recommended approach would be constrained by the limited nature of the trials. The long-term significance of any results would be questionable, since trials (by their very nature) are not the real world, and often prove to have limited applicability and success by the time promising trials are ready to be fully rolled out to the general population. Yet the systemic changes that could yield substantial efficiency gains are too big to be achieved in one big leap.

As the Productivity Commission rightly noted: "Implementing new payment models on a broader scale (including across all primary care, or over both primary and hospital care) would be more challenging, and would likely require larger-scale changes to the funding responsibilities of each level of government and private health insurance." [24] But the reality remains that trials have come and gone in the past, and led nowhere in terms of long-term reform. As the Grattan Institute has observed:

> Australia now has a considerable history of trials, pilots and demonstration projects investigating the introduction of chronic disease management in one form or another. These range from the ambitious coordinated care trials of the 1990s to the more recent Diabetes Care Project. But it has proved difficult to achieve major improvements in outcomes for chronic disease in the absence of broader change to the funding and organization of primary care and its relations to acute and extended care for regional populations.[25]

This poor track record of follow-through on trials may be the reason the Productivity Commission has also recommended an extended process-driven pathway to structural reform, supplemented by a "comprehensive review of the Australian health care system" that "could assess the potential benefits and costs of alternative payment models' draw lessons from past trials and international experience, and consult with relevant stakeholders."[26]

Trialling and testing, in combination with a holistic review, is the sum of what the Productivity Commission describes as reform process predicated on "steady and ongoing adjustment" as opposed to "abrupt and disruptive change."[27] Yet the benefits of a process-driven reform process are questionable, particularly less than a decade after the 2009 Final Report of the Rudd Government's National Health and Hospital Reform Commission (NHHRC). The expert-led NHHRC was established to advise the 'root-and-branch' reforms necessary to ensure the sustainability of the Australian health system in the twenty-first century. The NHHRC's major recommendation for long-term structural and payment reform was to advocate the replacement of Medicare with the Medicare Select model, which envisages all Australians receiving taxpayer-funded, risk-adjusted health insurance vouchers to fund the purchase of private health plans.

The rationale behind the Medicare Select proposal was to address the major structural problems with the current arrangements—as explained in Chapter 2. Individual health funds would hold the full financial risk for members' healthcare needs across the full service spectrum, and would operate as active purchasers of (instead of passive payers for) health services from providers competing to ensure patients receive the most appropriate and cost-effective care. Structural change on the insurance side of the Australian health system would in theory drive structural change on the services side of the system, and promote more efficient use of health resources.[28] However, the Medicare Select proposal—which is essentially the same model dubbed the 'Universal Service Obligation' by Private Health Australia—was not translated into policy action. This was in part because the NHHRC's reform 'blueprint' contained no political strategy to circumvent the institutional and cultural obstacles to implementation—a defect highly likely to feature in a report produced by an apolitical body such as the Productivity Commission.

A Modus Vivendi for Disruption

Despite the well-known defects and limitations of the rigid Medicare and regimented private insurance system, 'Big Bang' reforms of the existing architecture of the health system would entail enormous dislocations of current practice and carry the risk of unintended consequences. Fundamental changes to existing arrangements are also likely to be stymied equally well-known political obstacles regarding changes to Medicare.

What if there was a way to circumvent the impediments and avoid pitfalls of big bang reform, and minimize the inherent dangers of gambling $161 billion or the 10% of GDP spent annually on health on one big 'solution', but still allow for innovation — for disruption of established health payment and service delivery models — in a real world-applicable, commercial and competitive environment that would yield hard evidence far beyond trial quality, as well as establish governance and institutional structures that would support the case for scaling-up and for systemic reform?

There is a way to do all this is by establishing 'Health Innovation Communities' (HICs – see Box 3).

The idea of creating HICs is based on the concept of free trade zones that have been used throughout history to encourage commerce. The origins of free trade zones date back to the founding age of international trade. When eastern and western civilisations first started trading, free exchange of goods was facilitated by relaxing existing cultural norms and laws to the mutual benefit of both trading parties within strictly bounded areas to limit any unforeseen effects. In modern times, Free Trade Zones offered tax and other incentives to promote trade and development. Removing rigid rules, regulations and other disincentives that would otherwise impede new modes of doing business creates an 'ecosystem' in which innovation can flourish and percolate into the rest of the economy.

Drawing on these longstanding and successful examples, establishing 'free trade zones' for health innovation in Australia would be more than just another reform 'process'. Within the geographic areas declared to be HICs,

Box 3: Health Innovation Communities (HICs) – Key Design Specs

- Within geographic areas declared to be HICs, healthcare providers would apply for exemptions from existing health legislation and regulations to permit creation and use of alternative payment and service delivery models that are currently banned under Medicare and the *Health Insurance Act*.

- Companies, start-up entrepreneurs, charities, private health funds, and federal and state government health agencies would all be eligible to apply for registration as HIC-exempt providers by a joint government and industry-led HIC Commission.

- Exempt providers will accept and recruit individuals who want an alternative to the existing public and private health systems and who voluntarily choose to opt-in to an Integrated Care Plan (ICP). To prevent cream-skimming and a two-tiered system, a condition of the grant of exempt-provider status will be that ICPs must cater to both public and private patients; successful models will hereby be built fit for purpose, and be suitable for potential national, system-wide roll out under Medicare.

- ICPs will require inter-governmental and health sector agreements to 'pool' existing public and private sources of health funding (depending on the insurance status of each volunteer) on a capitation basis; a pooled funding model is essential to support genuinely integrated care, and give providers the ability, flexibility, and financial incentive to develop new, cost-effective care pathways.

- Appropriate safeguards will include a right for customers, when outside HICs, to access emergency care from traditional Medicare and private health insurance providers. Customers within HICs will also have the right to break the ICP service contract, and return to default Medicare and private insurance arrangements, in exceptional or egregious circumstances as arbitrated by an ICP Ombudsman. When ICP providers fail, consumers will also default back to Medicare, meaning no one will ever miss out on access to essential healthcare.

- HICs will be established in three to five areas to provide critical mass, benchmarking and competitive tension, and be allocated between the capital cities and also regional areas to ensure sufficient differentiation. Preferred locations will have proximity between a major hospital, university or medical school to support research, collaboration, training, measurement and control in partnership with Australia's renowned and world-leading publicly-funded medical research industry.

- Ideal sites will also have a target population base with high rates of obesity, chronic disease, and frequent use of hospital services related to chronic illness, and may include, for example, the catchment area for Westmead Hospital in Western Sydney, the Hunter region in mid-north coast of NSW, and the state of Tasmania.

healthcare providers could apply for exemptions from existing legislation to permit the creation of alternative payment and service models that are currently banned under Medicare and the *Health Insurance Act*. Companies, start-up entrepreneurs, charities, private health funds, federal government health agencies: the Primary Health Networks (PHNs) and state government health agencies: Local Hospital Districts (LHDs), would all be eligible to apply for registration as HIC-exempt providers of approved clinical services.

In effect, Medicare operates as an approved provider-captured statutory monopoly. Registered medical practitioners, who have been issued a Medicare provider number, are the only providers able to bill Medicare for professional attendances and other items listed on the MBS. A patient is not permitted by law to purchase a private health insurance policy where the insurer is liable to pay for patient services that would normally be payable under Medicare. Under Section 126 of the *Health Insurance Act*, a person is liable to be fined $1000 for entering mutually and freely into such an arrangement. Moreover, the *Private Health Insurance Act 2007* contains 334 pages of rules on private health insurance products, how insurers are to conduct their business. The maximum penalty for a fund offering a non-complying insurance product is a five-year prison sentence.[29] In essence, establishing HICs would make it legal for organisations, both public and private, to develop more efficient and sustainable models of care that would improve health outcomes. HICs would also make it legal for consumers to choose a publicly-funded alternative to the current structure of the Medicare scheme (the existing MBS benefits for GP and other medical and primary care services and right of access to free public hospital care) on an opt-in basis.

Within HICs, many different models would be able to be developed by a plurality of different providers offering different answers to the same problems. The discovery and knowledge-creation processes that would be unleashed would allow the proverbial '1000 flowers' to bloom—and to be simultaneously tested against each other—by releasing the existing structural and regulatory shackles on more innovative, efficient, and sustainable healthcare provision.

ICPs – Integrated Care Plans

Within HICs regions, exempt providers would be able to accept and recruit customers who seek an alternative to the existing public and private health insurance systems and who voluntarily choose to opt-in to an Integrated Care Plan (ICP). This would create a market for taxpayer-funded health services by giving consumers the option of choosing to leave the hitherto compulsory public system—and for funding to follow consumer choice.

ICPs will require inter-governmental and health sector agreements to pool existing funding (federal and state health funding, combined with private health funding—depending on the insurance status of each volunteer) on a per-capita basis in order to support an integrated, capitation-based funding model. Preliminary steps in this direction, away from strict fee-for-service remuneration, have already been taken with federal funding for the new $121 million chronic disease 'Health Care Home' trial to be provided on a quarterly capitation-basis in order to increase the range of allied health services, in addition to GP care, able to be purchased for patients who enrol with a general practice.[30]

However, a per-capita pool is not the only potential funding model that might be applied within HICs. One alternative would be to permit people across the socio-economic spectrum to contribute to the pool what they actually pay into or take out of the health system in the pursuit of securing superior services, better value for money, and, ultimately, premium reductions. For some individuals, this would be the value of their Medicare Levy and private health insurance premiums. For those reliant on government benefits, their contribution to the pool would be the amount of money calculated to normally be spent on their health care by the public system. Designing an individualised funding pool could open the way to including in the pool the individual funding available for people with disabilities under the National Disability Insurance Scheme.

Maximising the funding pool would enhance the chances of achieving early scale and increase the scope of innovations made possible, thereby raising the chances of longer term success of HICs, which would be jeopardised if ICP providers are under-capitalised at the outset. An important condition of granting exempt-provider status will be that ICPs must cater to both public and private patients. Privately insured patients would continue to have the option of choice of treatment in a private hospital. However, the requirement to enrol both public and private patients in ICPs will avoid cream-skimming and the creation of a two-tiered system, and will also mean that successful models will be built fit for purpose, and be suitable for potential national, system-wide roll out under Medicare.

Pooled funding (under any iteration) would give providers the ability, flexibility and financial incentive to develop more cost-effective ICPs. HICs would therefore allow for much more extensive funding and service innovation and integration. Under a pooled funding model, ICP providers will bear full financial responsibility for patient's entire health care needs, and will keep (or share) in the savings achieved, while being free to develop new care pathways that involve efficiencies and may incorporate novel services. For these reasons, HICs may provide an opportunity to revise the reinsurance arrangements for private health insurance. A system of prospective risk-adjusted payments based on the risk characteristics of fund members (as recommended by the 2013 National Commission of Audit)[31] could conceivably be added to the funding pool for ICPs.

Once freed from existing system-based cultural, institutional, and funding restrictions, providers would be free to include in their ICPs non-traditional services and incentives beyond standard clinical medical and hospital care. As well as managing utilisation by directing patients to lowest cost clinical settings, the real advantage ICP providers would have is the flexibility to fund and develop truly innovative preventive and chronic care plans involving novel care pathways that could reduce the disease burden, manage chronic illness more effectively, and minimise the use of high-cost hospital services. This could involve new behaviour change and social work-style services—perhaps coaching and financial incentives to change unhealthy lifestyles, or addressing the social problems (substance abuse, housing, employment, etc.) that make it hard for a low-income chronically ill person to self-manage their condition, receive full courses of treatment and access all appropriate and beneficial care. The existing service systems also provide no incentive, and limited assistance, for individuals to take responsibility for their own avoidable health risks. In the market environment created by HICs, we can anticipate providers drawing on the insights developed by the burgeoning field of behavioural economics. Research that informs about the incentives that work for different groups of people could potentially be applied to address the growing epidemic of 'lifestyle disease' in innovative and cost-effective ways — perhaps, for example, by using money, discounts, reward points, or concert or sport tickets to encourage obese people to lose weight or for diabetes sufferers to better control their blood glucose level. Similar upfront incentives could also be utilised to motivate patients to opt into ICPs.

Once the exemption was granted, PHNS, LHDs, and health funds may choose to develop their own 'in-house' ICPs. But — consistent with good public and private sector procurement practices — both health funds and government agencies may choose to develop a purchaser/provider split, and contract out service delivery to competing private sector health management companies that will develop their own models of care and virtual care networks by sub-contracting service delivery with GPs, specialists, hospitals, pharmacies, allied health, and other healthcare providers. This would also permit both government agencies and private funds to decide to give customers a choice of providers between competing ICP providers. This would facilitate the entry of new players into the health system, as well as giving established corporate primary care companies — whose business model currently relies on vertically integrating Medicare-funded GP, pathology and diagnostic imaging services — the opportunity to branch out into new areas of integrated care.

Private sector providers are also preferable — particularly start-ups — due to the risk management tools they will bring to evaluation and measurement of their services to demonstrate outcomes; creating a marketable value-proposition to sell to purchasers, and to ultimately produce returns for investors and shareholders. With regards to integrated care, non-traditional providers in other countries have innovated (and managed risk) by investment in information technology and data analysis to monitor service use, prevent duplication of tests and procedures through electronic medical records, and give feedback to clinicians and develop care protocols that achieve the best health outcomes. Investment in IT and analytics is where innovative providers are likely to seek to establish their competitive advantage.[32]

The new market-based system envisaged within HICs is not as radical as it sounds, given the precedent that exists. Under the Australian Defence Force's 'Garrison Health' contract, Medibank Private is responsible for organising the healthcare of all members of the ADF and for creating a 'preferred provider' network of medical, hospital and allied health services. A payment and service model that is good for the health of Australia's defence personnel would also be good for the health of many other Australians living in HICs. Parallels can also be drawn between the design and principles of HICs and the 'consumer-directed' reforms in the aged care sector (see Chapter 4).

Governance and Safeguards

HICs should number between three and five regions to provide critical mass, benchmarking and competitive tension, and be allocated between the capital cities and also regional areas to ensure sufficient differentiation. Ideal sites would have a target population base with high rates of obesity, chronic disease, and frequent use of hospital services related to chronic illness, and may include, for example, the catchment area for Westmead Hospital in Western Sydney, the Hunter region in mid-north coast of NSW, and, even, the state of Tasmania due to its geographic size and the location of its major health services concentrated in the cities of Hobart and Launceston.

Preferred locations would also have proximity between a major hospital, university or medical school to support research, collaboration, training, measurement and control. Australia's publicly-funded medical research sector, spread across teaching hospitals, the universities, and research institutes, is a renowned world-leader in the field. HICs would contribute to the growth of the sector by generating additional sources of research funding, as ICP providers will look to partner with leading research facilities to solve problems and measure and evaluate the performance and outcomes of their models. HICs will also be fertile territory for better 'bench-to-bedside', community and 'home-side' translation of medical research into innovative, evidence-based clinical practice via incorporation into ICPS to improve health outcomes, thereby addressing a defect—a longstanding failure to firmly embed the findings of medical research into the delivery of health care services—that was identified by the former CSIRO Chairman Simon McKeon's 2012 *Strategic Review into Health and Medical Research*. HICs would also be consistent with the McKeon review's recommendation that a more strategic approach to investment in medical research is required to improve the effectiveness and efficiency of Australian healthcare, and thus contribute to the health system sustainability by addressing the financial challenges posed in health by population ageing and the anticipated unaffordable increase in health costs in coming decades.[33]

Given that the fundamental objective of HICs is to encourage innovation, there is a need to ensure genuine flexibility and diversity in service provision by avoiding proscriptive regulation and administration as far as possible. This is particularly so when the intention is also to create a competitive and contestable environment for health service provision, in which the chief accountabilities will be determined by the market—by the ability to attract and keep customers enrolled in ICP programs, and secure service contracts from public or private purchasers. Part of the attraction of ICPs should be price competition for private insurance as customers see downward pressure on their premiums through provider success in improving the effectiveness of health care.

However, appropriate safeguards and oversight are needed. HICs would require a regulatory body or commission, whose joint, industry-led members would include representatives of the federal and state governments and health departments, the private health funds, and medical and consumer groups. The primary responsibility of the HIC Commission would be to vet and approve the registration of HIC exempt providers, and determine eligibility for access to pooled funding, based on appropriate clinical criteria consistent with the goal of access to universal healthcare.

Customers who sign up to ICPs would also need protections, such as a right to access emergency care when outside HICs from traditional Medicare and Private Health Insurance providers. Under these circumstances, it might be that the existing system absorbs these extraordinary costs for the sake of security and simplicity. However, the ICP provider could conceivably be required to cover these costs in fulfilment of a universal service obligation. In a mature market, it is likely that competitive HICs would develop provider relationships for their subscribers across the country or even overseas. However, apart from emergencies outside the HIC, strict rules would be needed to prevent doubling-dipping: a condition of signing up to an ICP would be to forfeit any right to traditional Medicare-funded services (either within or outside the HIC) for the duration of the contract. During that period, the commercial objective of the ICP provider would be to convince customers to renew their enrolment by providing a demonstrably superior service. Most importantly, however, customers within HICs would also have a right to break the ICP service contract, and return to default Medicare and private insurance arrangements, in exceptional or egregious circumstances. These circumstances may be stated upfront in the contract, as triggers for consumers to return to traditional payment and service arrangements. The right to default back to Medicare would also act as a safety net when ICP providers fail, meaning that consumers will never miss out on access to essential healthcare. The right of exit could also be protected and enforced by establishing the office of ICP Ombudsman. The Ombudsman would act as an honest broker and arbitrator for the resolution of disputes between providers and patients—and determine the financial consequences for providers that have failed to fulfil their end of the bargain, when patients leave due to bad experiences and the cost of their care is shifted back to Medicare.

Consumer groups—as well as medical bodies and other community organisations—could also play an important role within HICs by offering advocacy services. Such patient advocacy would be important not only in case of disputes, but to also help guide patients to appropriate ICPs, thus providing another layer of scrutiny and oversight to promote informed consumer choice and encourage providers to be responsive to consumer's needs.

Silicon Valleys for Health

Notwithstanding the necessary regulations and safeguards, the great advantage of HICs will be their superior agility as a means of incubating and developing good ideas into marketable health service products.

The founding principle of HICs—in stark distinction to the 'trial and test' model of service development that is the standard approach to reform and innovation within traditional healthcare systems—is the acknowledgment that no single entity, no single repository of collective wisdom, can come up with the complete solution to complex problems. Contrast the possibilities within HICs with the results of the existing trial-based approach. Take the federal government's $30 million, three-year Diabetes Care Project. Despite many promising elements—including investments in IT and data, quality payments linked to patient outcomes, flexible funding and funding for Care Facilitators — the evaluation showed the outcomes achieved and improvement in patient experience were not cost-effective.[34] And we are no further down the track to discovering what works—only what doesn't. In fact, the federal government is retracing its steps and has committed to another three-year $20 million trial of a fairly similar model.[35] While there is learning, and promising signs that can be taken away from each project, the cycle of periodic, serially-funded trials results in a very slow cycle of innovation, and the lack of follow through leading to systemic payment and service changes, and major improvements in chronic care outcomes, speak for themselves.

The problem with trials—along with the rigid program funding model that health departments employ in general—is that governments need to know what they are buying and paying for before they commit taxpayer's money to a particular model. But these top-down, rules-based, centrally-administered trials and programs that dictate all the things providers must do are the antithesis of the way real innovation occurs in the rest of the economy. Taxpayers end up paying for what is known will be done rather than paying for what actually works.[36] Achieving buy-in is also difficult, since providers, especially doctors, rationally calculate that it is not worthwhile re-inventing current practice in line with requirements that are likely to no longer apply after the end of the trial. HICs, by contrast, would create an environment in which innovations are generated from the bottom up, especially by entrepreneurial providers operating in a competitive and contestable market.

Technological advances are also revolutionising many aspects of the economy, including health. But if we are to discover alternative approaches quickly, apply the lessons rapidly, and realise the benefits in a timely fashion, we cannot linger over the current trial and test-based approach to incubating change. Given the lengthy periods of time such processes involve, and given the pace of change, the outcomes are liable to merely prove or disprove a model or advance that is already out of date. Outside the artificial confines of a trial, bad ideas and practices will be proven to have failed far quicker and will be weeded out, while successful ideas and practices will form the basis of further innovation—and guide investment decisions based on the risk management techniques that are standard in business but foreign to the health sector where strategic and operational decisions are guided by the availability of funding streams. Continuous innovation is essential – the kind of flexibility and adaptability that HICs would permit by creating an entire and constantly evolving industry founded on the pursuit of innovation. Each HIC would essentially constitute an Australian 'Silicon Valley' for health – hubs for research and development attracting the best and brightest to these locations to have the opportunity to create novel health products and solutions.

HICs would also allow competing models to be developed and results to be assessed simultaneously in parallel and real world settings. Commercially successful ICPs will be those developed by the providers that discover new and effective ways to deliver cost-effective and high-quality healthcare. These models will be marketable—they will be able to be sold to consumers, or funds, or government agencies—based on their demonstrated outcomes, initially within the HICs. Federal and state governments may also choose to roll out the best models outside the HICs by, for example, contracting a particular provider to manage the chronic care of patients within a certain local government or defined patient catchment area. Success would also give rise to export opportunities—HICs could potentially transform health from a drain on the public purse into a powerhouse of the national economy.

The comparison with Silicon Valley is especially apt given the significant potential for HICs to operate at the cutting edge of digital health innovation. As the Business Council of Australia has noted:

> Healthcare is reaching new levels of connectivity, automation and analysis. Leading providers are driving quality and efficiency with common technologies such as remote monitoring and clinical decision support, as well as next-generation innovations in analytics, genetic testing, 3D printing, etc. Consumers are being empowered to manage their own health and navigate the health system more effectively. They are adopting new tools such as online patient communities and fitness wearables, they are demanding care based on a universe of clinical information, and they are increasingly selective of providers and care plan. This affords new opportunities for innovative funding models to reward healthy behaviours, consumer education, and bottom-up momentum for change.[37]

Health is the last major sector to exploit data to improve customer focus and performance, but this is changing. Global advances in health informatics, such as at the UK's Farr Institute,[38] are inspiring investment, albeit uneven, in some leading Australian health provider communities. HICs could catalyse further health data science investment in diagnosis and therapy, and use real time analytics to make best use of resources. The potential of health informatics could be further unlocked if HIC providers shared their data with a mutually incentivised public system. The United States government's open source health data program—which "has resulted in an explosion of patient and provider focused applications and technologies"—could serve as the model for HICs to gain access to existing local stores big data.[39]

What HICs Is and Is *Not* Advocating

To ensure the key principles and purposes of Health Innovation Communities are not misinterpreted, it is important to clarify what this research report is and is *not* advocating.

The shift from fee-for-service payments to a capitation-based model that is envisaged may create the false impression that HICs will simply create an environment in which the Medicare Select idea can be trialled and tested. This impression could also be created by the fact that individuals opting-in to ICPs will have their healthcare provided by a 'fund-holding' organisation that will function as the 'insurer' or 'payee' covering medical expenses. However, the obvious point of difference between HICs and Medicare Select is that private health insurance funds will not be the sole fund-holders as Medicare Select would entail. Instead, within HICs, a range of public, NGO and private providers will be free to gain HIC-exempt status and compete as ICP providers, including, most crucially, new entrants into the market—start-ups firms that will introduce genuinely innovative thinking and new service models into the health sector. This is the crucial difference: whereas Medicare Select is conceived of as the 'One Big Solution' for the structural problems in the health system, HICs, by clear and absolute contrast, are not the solution but are rather the first step to creating the environment in which solutions can be proposed and refined *at the coal-face of patient care and service delivery.*

The Medicare Select model also envisages general risk pooling via a taxpayer-payer funded, risk-rated insurance premium payment mechanism—a 'voucher system' that would be portable and would follow customers to their private health fund of choice. Under these arrangements, health funds would assume responsibility for managing the care of all members—regardless of how costly or complex that care is. However, HICs are designed instead to use financial incentives and financially accountable delivery of health services to spur the discovery of more effective ways to reorganise the complex and costly care of the estimated 5-10% of chronic patients who suffer multiple comorbidities. Those 'frequent flyers' whose care is estimated to account for approximately 50% of total health spending, and who are readily identifiable and thus will able to be targeted by ICP providers will be encouraged to opt-in through strategies including use of upfront incentives.

Misleading comparisons could also be drawn to the health reform agenda of the Obama administration in the United States. The US Medicare Innovation program implemented under the *Affordable Care Act* permits Accountable Care Organisations (ACOs) to apply to the federal government's 'Medicare and Medicaid Services Innovation Center' to participate in tests and trials of "innovative payment and service delivery models to reduce program expenditures."[40] The parallels with the HIC concept might appear obvious, but more important are the key differences. American ACOs must apply to the Innovation Center to gain approval of a pre-determined model of care that will be subject to evaluation. This top-down approach essentially entails a bureaucracy centrally-planning a series of new programs, which consist of rules-based, centrally-administered protocols that dictate all the things that providers must do.

For the reasons explained in the previous chapter, the ACO model of 'innovation' is demonstrably flawed in conception and execution because the proper roles that ought to be played by buyers and sellers of goods and services are confused in bureaucratic health systems. "Successful innovations are produced by entrepreneurs, *challenging* conventional thinking—not by bureaucrats *trying to implement* conventional thinking." In the case of chronic care services, "buyers of a product (i.e. health bureaucrats) are trying to tell the sellers how to efficiently produce it."[41] The fact that compliance with bureaucrat mandates stymies real innovation helps to explain why the available evidence (examined in Chapter 2) shows that government-operated 'coordinated care' programs have been ineffective.[42] To give but one example, the flagship, multi-million dollar NSW Health Chronic Disease Management Program targeted 'frequent flying' chronic disease patients; but despite implementing a range of new protocols and services coordinating the care of these patients, the 2014 evaluation showed the anticipated reductions in hospital admission had not occurred.[43]

The top-down approach to health innovation also means consumers are left to take what they are given by the government agencies, with little choice of alternatives. Real innovation in the rest of the economy is generated from the bottom up: entrepreneurs operating in competitive environments discover new, better, and lower cost ways to deliver services to consumers who are free to choose between competing providers based on quality and price. HICs recognise, and are specifically designed to lift, the dead-hand of command-and-control rigidities over the production of health services. The rigidities that mar the health sector will be avoided due to the light regulatory framework that is proposed. Consistent with sound regulatory principles, the regulatory impact of the HIC Commission and Ombudsman will be targeted squarely at dealing with bad performers rather than focused on micro-managing good performers. HICs will therefore create, as far as possible and practical, a flexible environment that replicates the dynamic and innovation-spurring features of efficient and competitive markets.

Another key difference with the HIC concept is that ICP providers will be required to include performance measurement and evaluations in their model of care, rather than be subject to external evaluation by government agencies as per the standard test and trial regime. Measurement of outcomes is standard practice in the private sector in order to justify business cases, inform rational decisions about resource allocation, and maintain and add to shareholder value. Performance measures and evaluation data will also be an important way for ICP providers to market their services to consumers, who will be empowered both by the freedom to choose their provider and by the information publicly available about competing providers.

Bi-Partisan Health Reform

Given the 2016 'Mediscare' federal election, it might appear a bad time to be proposing health reforms of any description. The political challenges are reinforced by recalling the 2015 Queensland state election, where the health reform agenda of the Newman government contributed to the electoral disaster that befell the Liberal National Party and returned the Labor Party to office after just three years in the political wilderness.

Yet it is state governments—regardless of whether they are of Labor or Coalition stripe—that stand to benefit from working with the federal government to create solutions to the health policy puzzle. Health expenditure accounts for between 25% to 33% of total state government expenditure, and the ever-rising cost of health is acknowledged as the major source of fiscal pressure and the major threat to the long-term sustainability of state budgets.

States ought therefore to look favourably on the HIC proposal, which would allow state governments to reap the financial rewards that would flow from achieving more cost-effective health service provision. A state, for example, state governments—which routinely seek to restructure state health and hospital systems[44]—should welcome the HIC concept, not only due to the financial benefits of reducing avoidable hospital admissions. HICs would also address a long-running sore point within the federation by permitting the federal government's 'own program' health expenditure to be directly applied and more effectively deployed to address state government's health expenditure and service delivery challenges.

Fiscal bribes—federal 'incentive payments' to the states—ought not be needed to get states to commit to the HICs. But financial inducements may be a necessary evil to make states act rationally in their own best interest. Regardless of this, uptake of the HIC proposal ultimately depends on genuine political leadership at both state and federal levels to rise above the populism and 'magic pudding' attitudes that have unfortunately dominated the health debate in recent times. State government buy-in to the objectives of HICs will also be essential to help ameliorate the potentially fatal squabbling that negotiation and calculation of state and federal contributions to the capitation funding pool will inevitably involve.

Releasing the Shackles on Innovation

It is widely recognised that the growth of the Australian economy in the twenty-first century will depend on our ability to develop high-skill, value-adding industries. Without innovation—unless our resources are used more wisely and productively to create the goods and services we need and want—the living standards and wellbeing of all Australians will suffer. The same fundamental principles of economic reform need to apply to health, given the large and ever-increasing proportion of the nation's income (near 10% of GDP) consumed by health, and the deleterious financial and other consequences of continuing to do our health business as usual in a less than efficient—and ultimately unsustainable—fashion.

Given the financial challenges posed by the ever-escalating cost of health to government budgets, we must start somewhere to catalyse change. The report of the 2013 National Commission of Audit described health spending as the "single largest long-run fiscal challenge." The report went on to state that:

> Australia's health system is not equipped to face these future challenges and a universal health scheme is unlikely to be sustained without reform. We need to make the system we have work better. Putting health care on a sustainable footing will require reforms to make the system more efficient and competitive. The supply of health services must increase in line with growth in demand and improvements in productivity are a natural way of ensuring this. More deregulated and competitive markets, with appropriate safeguards, have the greatest potential to improve the sector's competitiveness and productivity...[T]here are no instant or easy solutions to the challenges of health care. But we should be prepared to take steps now to begin strengthening the health system, otherwise more difficult and painful reforms will be needed later.[45]

Structural health reforms could release billions of health dollars that are currently locked up in the rigid Medicare and regimented private health systems. The financial prize is large; but so are the political, institutional, and cultural walls protecting the vested interests of stakeholders with privileged access to the 'rents' generated by the existing health regulatory regimes. More efficient providers of healthcare need to have an opportunity to compete for this money in a market environment.

Health reform would return a dividend to the community not only in the form of higher-quality and more cost-effective health services, but also by releasing resources to pay for additional health services, or to fund other areas of government activity, or to cut taxes and increase private income and wealth. Individuals would benefit financially, and in terms of health and wellbeing, from innovations that not only lower the cost of health to government and the cost of private insurance, but also reallocate and use resources more efficiently to improve health outcomes. The trouble with health reform is that the changes that are needed to deliver highly desirable innovations are too big to be imminently achievable; hence we need to focus on reforms that are possible as opposed to optimal but unattainable.

Health Innovation Communities are a viable and creative way of taking steps now to disrupt the existing system — their creation would mark a real step towards addressing the future challenges we face in health, by initiating the reform process in a competitive and market environment. Allowing health funds to control benefit outlays by purchasing more efficient services is crucial at a time when spiralling use of insured services is driving rises in premiums and threatens to make private health insurance unaffordable for consumers. The service gaps, out-of-pocket expenses, and stress, frustration and bewilderment many chronic disease patients experience in navigating a fractured and complex health system are well-known, and the multiple band-aids that have been applied over many years have failed to heal this long-weeping sore. HICs will not only benefit individuals financially by lowering the cost of health to government and the cost of private insurance. HICs will, for the first time, put the needs of chronic patients at the centre of the health system, as cost-effective ICPs are developed that provide continuity of care and ensure chronic patients receive the full cycle of all necessary care to properly manage and maintain their conditions.

The potential outcomes of HICs should also be compared with the prospects of the Turnbull government's health policy. The Medical Benefits Schedule Review Taskforce, which has identified a number of rorts, wasteful and inefficient MBS items, is another band-aid that fails to adequately address the fundamental systemic issues. The as yet uncosted savings generated by the MBS Review, which will in theory offset cost of the Health Care Home trial, are certain to be relatively puny compared to the scale of potential savings—the estimated $17 billion annual net welfare loss due to inefficiencies across the health system—that could be achieved through innovative integration of services.[46] The federal government should embrace HICs as a way of harnessing the creativity and initiative of non-government organisations and as a means of helping the private sector to help solve the government's intractable problems in health.

A national health innovation policy that establishes HICs can ameliorate the toxic, innovation-killing politics of health. The current Medicare entitlements and private health insurance arrangements of the vast majority of the population, and the familiar public and private payment and service systems, will remain intact, with exemptions from the existing rules only applying within HIC-declared regions. Moreover, ICPs will apply only to those consumers who live within HICs and who choose to opt-in to the alternative system. These are the answers to the inevitable scare campaign the public health lobby and other defenders of the status quo will mount of the 'thin edge of the wedge' variety, and by claiming HICs are a wholesale attack on Medicare. Such claims are inherently false, of course. HICs will maintain the core principles of fairness at the heart of Medicare—that is: taxpayer-funded, equitable access to high quality and affordable health services for all Australians, irrespective of means.

Critics also need to understand that healthcare innovation is currently occurring; albeit in a limited and piecemeal fashion—and with access to new models of care determined solely by income. Those who can afford to self-fund their care can already avail themselves of privately-operated aged care and chronic disease services. Those with higher incomes can thus pay to receive integrated care and assistance to navigate the fragmented private and public health systems. [47] HICs would help stem the development of the much-feared two-tiered health system by making these kind of services available to patients regardless of income, and funded entirely from the public purse.

Another likely scare tactic will be allegations that 'rich corporates' will cut services to make money at patients' expense. This not only ignores the important safeguards built into the HIC design, but also the media scrutiny that such a high-profile experiment in healthcare innovation will generate. Providers will be acutely aware of the reputational risks—and risk to shareholder value—of failing to satisfy customer needs. In the new market environment, moreover, the success or failure of the new models of care developed in HICs will ultimately depend on the quality of patient experience provided, and thus the ability of ICP providers to attract and retain customers.

Finally, HICs will not threaten the primacy or principles of Medicare. The HIC concept questions the current fee-for-service Medicare arrangements; and especially its GP-centric approach to primary care, given its well-recognised limitations in addressing chronic diseases and preventative health. However, the concept also affirms the core principle of fairness at the heart of Medicare—universal availability of affordable, taxpayer-funded healthcare for all citizens—under the new and potentially diverse payment and service models foreshadowed here as emerging within Health Innovation Communities.

Public subsidies for health will continue to provide equitable access to health services, and no Australian will go without healthcare due to lack of income. However, HICs will allow those living within their boundaries to choose an alternative form of healthcare provision, and allow for new ways to be developed to use our increasingly scarce health dollars to provide better and more sustainable health services to Australians. The opportunities HICs will open up for payment and service innovations will, however, demonstrate the benefits of doing things differently in health to achieve more efficient and cost-effective services. The good examples and real world (as opposed to trial quality) evidence of better practice and outcomes that will be rapidly generated will seed structural reform by establishing functioning models and workable blueprints for systemic—and sustainable—change. The superior financial results achieved, combined with the improved outcomes for patients, could potentially create broader community consensus and support for releasing the shackles on innovative models of healthcare payment and service delivery across the entire health system.

Endnotes

1   Health Reform: Higher Quality, Lower Costs. A Port Jackson Partners Limited Report to Private Healthcare Australia, May 2014, 11.

2   OECD Reviews of Health Care Quality: Australia 2015: http://www.oecd.org/australia/oecd-reviews-of-health-care-quality-australia-2015-9789264233836-en.htm

3   Productivity Commission, Efficiency in Health, Research Paper, (Canberra: 2015), 34.

4   Jeremy Sammut, Medi-Value: health insurance and service innovation in Australia - implications for the future of Medicare, Research Report 14, (Sydney: The Centre for Independent Studies, 2016).

5   Productivity Commission, Efficiency in Health, 95.

6   Productivity Commission, Efficiency in Health, 2.

7   Sammut, Medi-Value.

8   Productivity Commission, Efficiency in Health, 34.

9   Productivity Commission, Efficiency in Health, 9.

10 Sammut, Medi-Value.

11 David Gadiel, Towards a More Competitive Medicare: The Case for Deregulating Medical Fees and Co-payments in Australia, Research Report 1, (Sydney: The Centre for Independent Studies, 2015).

12 The authors are grateful to an informed reviewer with knowledge of private health systems on both sides of the Tasman for pointing this out.

13 Productivity Commission, Efficiency in Health, 63-7.

14 Sammut, Medi-Value.

15 Productivity Commission, Efficiency in Health, 66-67.

16 'Medibank plays hardball over hospital "mistakes"', The Australian (21 July,, 2015).

17 Health Reform: Higher Quality, Lower Costs, 3, 5-6.

18 Productivity Commission, Efficiency in Health, 1

19 Private Healthcare Australia, Submission: Private Health Insurance Consultations 2015-16, 3.

20 Medibank Private, Improving private health for consumers through transparency, affordability and value, December 2015, 2-3.

21 Health Reform: Higher Quality, Lower Costs, 7.

22 Health Reform: Higher Quality, Lower Costs, 35, 50.

23 Productivity Commission, Efficiency in Health, 3, 70.

24 Productivity Commission, Efficiency in Health, 39.

25 Hal Swerissen and Stephen Duckett, Chronic Failure in Primary Care, Grattan Institute Report No. 2016-2, March 2016. 22.

26 Productivity Commission, Efficiency in Health, 39.

27 Productivity Commission, Efficiency in Health, 95.

28 Sammut, Medi-Value, 2.

29 Section 84.1, Private Health Insurance Act, 2007.

30 Better Outcomes for People with Chronic and Complex Health Conditions, Report of the Primary Health Care Advisory Group, December 2015.

31 National Commission of Audit, Towards Responsible Government, (Australian Government: Canberra, 2014), 101.

32 Sammut, Medi-Value, 20.

33 Strategic Review of Health and Medical Research in Australia, (Australian Government: Canberra, 2012).

34 Evaluation Report of the Diabetes Care Project, (Canberra: Australian Government, 2015).

35 http://www.health.gov.au/internet/ministers/publishing.nsf/Content/health-mediarel-yr2016-ley024.htm

36 Sammut, Medi-Value, 13.

37 Business Council of Australia, Overview of Megatrends in Health and their Implications for Australia, Background Paper, (BCA: Melbourne 2015). 2-3

38 http://www.farrinstitute.org/

39 Business Council of Australia, Overview of Megatrends in Health, 14 18.

40 https://innovation.cms.gov/About/index.html

41 John C. Goodman, Priceless: Curing the Healthcare Crisis, (The Independent Institute: Oakland, 2012), 73-4.

42 Sammut, Medi-Value.

43 State-Wide Evaluation NSW Chronic Disease Management Program, Final Report, October 2014: http://www.health.nsw.gov.au/cdm/Documents/CDMP-Evaluation-Report-2014.pdf

44 Jeremy Sammut, 'The way to get more hospital care and reduce waiting times is to close down public hospitals', Adelaide Advertiser, 2 March, 2015.

45 National Commission of Audit, Towards Responsible Government, 95-6.

46 'Sweeping Medicare changes to curb rorts', The Australian, 12 September, 2016.

47 https://www.nationalcaremanagement.com.au/about; http://www.relianthealthcare.com.au/

Chapter 4

Consumer-Directed Aged Care[*]

Jeremy Sammut

A Shining Example

The 'consumer-directed' aged care (CDC) reforms are of the most important sets of reforms to Australia's human services sector in a generation. They are of great significance, given that Australian governments are generally struggling to achieve the equally necessary consumer-focused, market-based and sustainable reform in other areas of large public spending across the human services sectors. Aged care (along with disability services) is one of the few human services sectors in which the principles and recommendations of the 2015 Harper Competition Policy Review have started to be implemented. The Harper Review highlighted the need for governments to undertake reforms that place consumer choice at the centre of service delivery, combined with regulatory changes that maximise choice and competition, encourage diversity in provision, foster innovation in service delivery and drive improvements in efficiency.[1]

The genesis and implementation of the CDC system also teach important lessons about how the process of reform can be driven from the grass roots, and help policymakers transcend the political obstacles to change in government-funded service sectors. At a time of considerable pessimism in the Australian community about the ability of governments to achieve structural reforms in important areas of the national economy, it is worth examining a positive story of policy change and pondering the lessons. Understanding 'how' the CDC reforms were implemented is thus as

---

[*] First published as Real Choice for Ageing Australians: Achieving the Benefits of the Consumer-Directed Aged Care Reforms in the New Economy, Research Report 24, (Sydney: The Centre for Independent Studies, 2017).

important as 'why' they were implemented. This is crucial in terms of trying to emulate similar reforms in other government service sectors facing similar policy, cost and service delivery challenges, including the health sector. Given that Medicare is essentially a provider-captured payment system, which locks consumers into traditional GP-led or hospital-based healthcare delivery systems—and prevents the development of innovative, more cost-effective alternative models of care—there is much to learn from the way the CDC reforms have addressed the same issues in relation to aged care services. [2]

With regard to the broader challenges of structural reform, and given the tight budgetary situation confronting both federal and state governments, the major lesson to be drawn from the CDC reforms is how better performance—more and better quality government-funded services with minimal additional public cost, plus greater private investment in service delivery[3]—can be achieved by ensuring that government funding is spent in the most efficient and effective ways. The imperative to limit the call on public resources and maximise the outcomes achieved for the funding expended—without resort to the so-called 'solution' of simply spending more taxpayers' money—is especially vital in a fiscally sensitive area such as aged care, where demand and expenditure will grow rapidly in line with the ageing of the population.[4] The need for the CDC reforms to generate better value for limited funding was reinforced by the cuts to aged care funding announced as part of the 2016 federal budget.[5]

A New Era for Aged Care Services

The Consumer-Directed Care (CDC) reforms came into full effect on 27 February, 2017. On that date, all 'Home Care Packages' started to follow consumers and became completely portable. Home care packages are the taxpayer-funded subsidy provided by the federal government to give people assessed as having complex and multiple ageing-related needs access to home-based care and support services to enable them to live safely and well in their own homes. Home-based aged care services include the Commonwealth Home Support Program that provides entry-level support

Figure 3: Aged Care in Australia

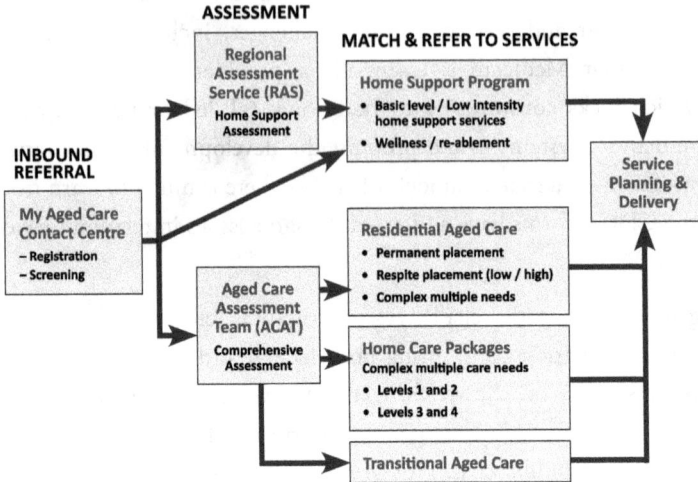

(including assistance with cleaning and meals); home care packages, now CDC packages, are designed to provide access to more intensive care and support for people with needs ranging from basic to high needs (Figure 3)

The introduction of fully portable home care packages means ageing Australians have for the first time been empowered with the freedom to choose the type and mix of home-based aged care services they wish to receive, and have been given the freedom to choose the service provider they prefer.

The implementation of full portability has completed the funding reforms implemented on 1 July, 2015. From that date, all funding for home care packages was converted into CDC packages that replaced the long-established system of bulk funding of 'Approved Providers' who—having undergone a competitive vetting process to be eligible to provide care—were contracted by public tender to deliver a set quantity of packages within specific geographic regions for which they received per package payments from the federal government. In place of this highly-regimented 'supply-driven" (and ultimately provider-captured) regime, the new demand-driven system allows ageing Australians requiring home care to access individualised funding budgets to purchase the care they require based on personal choice. (Figure 4)

The amount of CDC funding an individual receives is tiered across four increments according to level of need. The level is assessed by the Aged Care Assessment Team (ACAT), the federal government agency that employs health and medical professionals to determine eligibility for subsidised aged care services. A means test (effective from 1 July 2014) was also introduced as part of the CDC reforms, and takes the form of mandatory income-related 'co-payments' that are paid out-of-pocket by individuals.[6] (Figure 5)

In the transition phase from the old to the new system, consumer choice was constrained by continuing government regulation. Consumers still had to accept packages that were available and 'held' (won by tender) by approved providers. On 27 February, the legacy restrictions on choice were abolished, and consumers holding a CDC package are now free to choose their provider. Approved providers will continue (for administrative purposes) to hold and manage funding on behalf of, and at the direction, of consumers. But instead of having to receive a full service from the approved provider, consumers are now free to choose an alternative provider, and determine the kind of care and support they want from their preferred provider.

The CDC reforms are designed to give consumers greater control over the design and delivery of their care by transforming their role from passive recipients into empowered, active purchasers of home care services. The old funding system essentially allowed providers to 'capture' the system and dictate the overall cost and service delivery outcomes achieved. Under the old system, the consumer's choice of type and mix of services was limited to the kind of one-size-fits-all service model the provider chose to deliver. Under the new system, consumers will no longer depend on traditional providers or be obliged to 'take what they are given'.

Hence, a key objective of the CDC reforms is to ensure that elderly Australians have choice and control over what, how, and when they receive the kinds of services that best allow them to 'age in place' for as long as possible in their own homes, and delay the need to move to higher cost (for both governments and consumers) residential aged care facilities.[7] The introduction into the home care sector of consumer choice and provider competition is intended to drive improvements in the quality and cost of care. Providers seeking to win the custom of those who are free to take their business elsewhere will now have to be aware of the needs of customers in order to compete successfully. The old system did not allow for the personalising of services according to the diverse needs, expectations and preferences of today's more demanding consumers, especially among the ageing baby boomer demographic who are assisting ageing parents receiving care, or in the early stages of accessing care themselves. In the new dynamic market-based environment, the benefits of choice and competition are expected to include tailoring or personalising the range of services offered to care recipients' individual needs and preferences, and spur providers to discover operational efficiencies and other innovations that will increase the amount and/or mix of services that can be delivered from the funding package. The aim of the CDC model is to put consumers (instead of providers) at the centre of the system, generate better value for current and future taxpayers' money by promoting efficient service delivery, and ensure elderly Australians in need receive more—and higher quality—services for the available funding.

Given the broader implications of the CDC reforms, this chapter seeks to identify the potential barriers to their success. The point stressed is that the CDC system could fall short of its promise—as measured by failing to optimise the potential outcomes for consumers, care workers, governments and taxpayers—due to lack of follow-up and follow-through reforms to remove other regulatory barriers. This is to say that consumer-directed aged care could prove less successful than hoped, not because the reforms 'go too far' but because they don't go far enough to yield the full benefits for the recipients, providers and funders of home-based aged care. The policy recommendations herein (see Box 4) encourage the federal government to implement a range of additional reforms to promote real choice and greater improvements in the efficiency and effectiveness of consumer-driven aged care in the new economy.

Figure 4: From Supply-Driven to Consumer-Driven

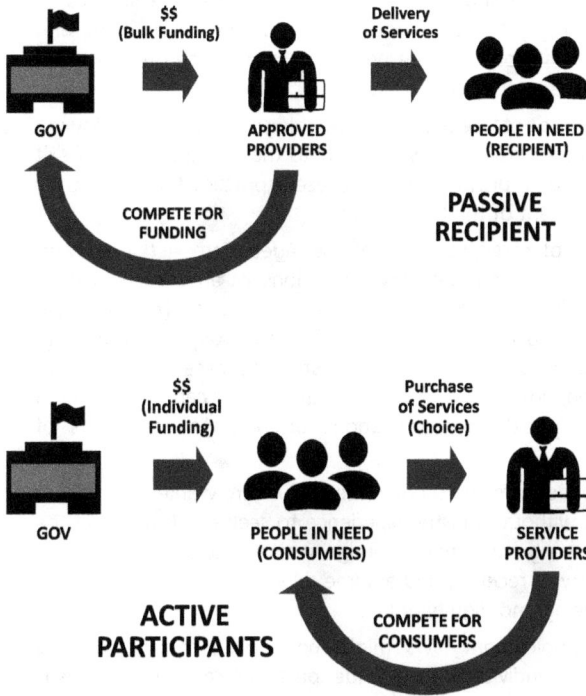

Figure 5: Home Care Package

Level of home care package	Home care subsidy rates		Maximum daily contribution based on income		
	Per annum	Per day	income < $26,327.60 p.a	income $26,327.60 to $50,876.80 p.a	income > $50,876.80 p.a
Level 1	$8,157.75	$22.35	$10.17	$14.59*	$29.19**
Level 2	$14,837.25	$40.65	$10.17	$14.59*	$29.19**
Level 3	$32,620.05	$89.37	$10.17	$14.59*	$29.19**
Level 4	$49,592.55	$135.87	$10.17	$14.59*	$29.19**

*Annual cap of $5,313.28 per year for part pensioners, **Annual cap of $10,626.59 per year for self-funded retirees
Lifetime Cap of $63,759.75 for all income-tested care fees, including residential care fees
Note: Amounts increase on 20 March & 20 September each year in line with aged pension increases.
Source: Australian Government Department of Health, accessed November 2017.

> **Box 4. Aged Care Reform 'To Do' List**
>
> - Establish a minimum standards framework for home care services to ensure excessive regulation does not restrict provider competition—and therefore customer choice—in the new consumer-focused market, and doesn't burden the sector with excessive cost.
>
> - Ensure consumers do not face significant switching costs, by foreshadowing the application of Australian consumer law to the charging of hefty exit fees should traditional providers fail to cease a practice that is contrary to the spirit and intent of the CDC reforms.
>
> - Review the duty of care provisions of the *Aged Care Act* to prevent traditional providers citing statutory obligations as an excuse to deny consumers the right to choose alternative providers. This will help stimulate the unbundling of one-size-fits-all care packages into separate services (spanning fund holding, administration, case management, care coordination, advocacy and service delivery) that can be purchased discretely from specialised organisations offering different parts of the bundle.
>
> - Revisit mandatory qualification requirements for care workers to make it easier for those without industry experience to seek employment in the sector, while trusting consumers to judge workers' suitability based on the quality of service received and assume a level of risk consistent with independent ageing and dignity of life.
>
> - Examine how employment laws might be applied to an individual engaging another individual to provide personal care and domestic service, to clarify the status of care workers as independent contractors hired directly by consumers. This will encourage the growth of innovative online marketplaces for care and support services that can offer better value and superior quality home care.
>
> - Undertake a public information education campaign to foster awareness among ageing Australians and care recipients of their right to choose under the CDC system, and promote knowledge of the full range of options now available, including online platforms.

Background: Consumer-Focused, Bi-Partisan Reform

In April 2010, the Rudd Government instructed the Productivity Commission to inquire into Australia's aged care sector.[8] The inquiry was sparked in part by the Government's recent commitment to take over full funding and policy responsibility for the disability and aged care sector (as part of the establishment of the NDIS—the National Disability

Insurance Scheme). However, the inquiry—as was ultimately reflected in the findings and recommendations of the Productivity Commission's final report—was also prompted by mounting concerns and frustrations expressed by consumers, families and advocacy groups about the inability of the existing, largely inflexible and high-cost aged care system to respond to significant shifts in the type of aged care being demanded by increasing numbers of elderly Australians who preferred independent living arrangements and to live in their own homes. Policymakers were also motivated by an awareness that the current system was ill-equipped to meet the increasing demand for services in a rapidly ageing Australia, and that among the most important challenges was the need to expand the size (and improve the wages and conditions) of the aged care workforce.

A month later, in May 2010, the Henry tax review (*Australia's Future Tax System Review*[9]) was released and made specific recommendations relating to aged care services. The review recommended less regulation of the sector and found there was "considerable scope to align aged care assistance with the principles of user-directed funding to provide assistance in line with recipients' needs." The report advised the Productivity Commission to consider recommending reforms along these lines, together with appropriate regulatory changes.[10]

In August 2011, the Productivity Commission released its final report, *Caring for Older Australians*.[11] The report found the sector struggled with a number of weaknesses, including: consumers having limited choice, receiving limited services and limited coverage of needs; difficulties accessing information and navigating complex assessment and funding arrangements; uneven quality of care; and inconsistent or inequitable pricing and subsidies. The Commission proposed an "integrated package of reforms" to tackle the major structural challenges facing the sector, and made the following recommendations:

- Establish a new regulatory agency, the Australian Aged Care Commission, to ensure independent governance and regulation of standards.
- Create a single, simplified online gateway to access aged care services and information.

- Establish a means test for co-contributions and a lifetime limit of co-contributions.
- Replace the current care package regime with a single system of integrated and flexible care provision to increase consumer choice, access and financial sustainability.

In April 2012, in response to the Productivity Commission report, the Gillard Government unveiled the *Living Longer, Living Better* aged care reform package.[12] The proposed reforms were welcomed and garnered initial support across the sector. Due to support and lobbying by consumer advocacy groups such as COTA Australia, the *Living Longer, Living Better* package enjoyed bi-partisan support in Parliament. Following extensive consultation with the community, there was broad-based political acknowledgement of the need for change, and both the government and the opposition saw the merit of putting the care of older Australians and the needs of consumers, their families and taxpayers ahead of the "business imperatives" of traditional providers with vested interests in the status quo.[13]

The legislation implementing the Aged Care Reform Package passed in June 2013, and introduced the following changes:

- Established the Aged Care Pricing Commission, Aged Care Quality Agency, and Aged Care Financing Authority.
- Created a new, simplified gateway, the My Aged Care website, with easily accessible information, screening and needs assessments.
- Increased residential care places by 29,500, and home care packages by 40,000 over 5 years.
- Introduced fairer and more transparent, means-tested thresholds and tiers for co-contributions, including the introduction of a $60,000 lifetime limit on co-contributions.
- Replaced bulk funding of home care packages with individualised CDC funding packages.

The fundamental reforms announced by the Gillard Government were largely based on the Productivity Commission's recommendations, and were set to be implemented progressively over three years to allow for a smooth transition. The reforms aimed, in the first instance, to reorganise the governance of the system and to increase the amount of recurrent government investment in aged care by expanding the number of packages available. The ratio of home care to residential care funding packages was increased, and funding for home care packages was also substantially increased. However, the additional 'investment' in the sector was a canny one in concert with the introduction of the CDC system. Rather than simply add additional funding 'inputs', the overall objective was to increase 'outputs': the quantity and range of services delivered from available funding by putting consumers in charge of their care and spurring competition, innovation and efficiency among providers.

Reorienting the system around consumers began with the establishment of the My Aged Care gateway to provide consumers with better and more easily accessible information about their rights and options available, as is standard policy when governments undertake market-based reforms. But the major step in the consumer-focused direction was, of course, the move to CDC packages, with the aim being to wrest control of service design and delivery away from traditional providers by empowering consumers with the right to choose their own levels of support and services.

Objectives: More Care, Better Quality

Under the old, supply-driven funding system, the federal government purchased home care services in bulk from providers who determined the model of care—the type and mix of services provided. The paternalistic relationship established between providers and consumers probably derives from the 'charitable' status of the Not-For Profit, usually faith-based organisations that dominate the sector, among the over 2000 aged care service providers in Australia supplying both residential and home-based services.[14]

From colonial times, Australian governments have subsidised the work of voluntary organisations providing assistance to the poor and vulnerable. The work of these charitable bodies, which were mostly controlled by churches, included the provision of homes ("asylums") for the aged.[15] These institutions were the forerunners of today's 'nursing homes'.[**] The inflexible, one-size-fits-all, impersonal nature of the home-based services delivered by many traditional providers resembles an 'institutionalised' model of care—but without the walls. This model of care is underpinned by well-intentioned assumptions about providers knowing what is best for 'vulnerable' elderly care recipients—assumptions that can ultimately feel patronising and ageist because they fail to take into account and reflect the capacity of many elderly people to make informed decisions about their care needs and service requirements. As the Aged Care Reform Implementation Council chair Peter Shergold observed, "the problem is that even with good intentions ... [at] every forum I've attended in which consumers have had a voice, they excoriate providers who are perceived to patronise them."[16] This issue—and hence the need to empower consumers with greater choice and control — was highlighted by the Productivity Commission's *Caring for Older Australians* report, which recommended a more reasonable and balanced approach to choice and risk be applied across the sector as a part of the CDC reforms (see 'Risk' below).

Whatever its historical roots, provider-driven home care has impeded the development of responsive and innovative service delivery. The service provider market has historically been dominated by Approved Providers that are mostly similar organisations offering similar standardised sets of services and service delivery terms to consumers denied any real alternatives. The rigidities within the traditional care model also stem from operational considerations pertaining to centralised rostering of the care worker workforce by head office managers. Rotating rostered staff in and out of homes to undertake set tasks in a set time frame—in effect delivering an 'institutionalised'-style service—does not allow for the personalising of services according to the diverse needs, expectations and preferences of today's more demanding consumers. Nor does it allow for consumers to have the basic right of privacy and to control who comes into their homes.

The historic, hierarchical structure of traditional home care services also reinforces perceptions of care and support workers being a low-skilled, poorly-paid profession, thereby exacerbating retention and recruitment challenges. This rigid structure also inhibits the human dimensions of care — the development of a personal relationship between care worker and consumer that is vital to worker morale and the recipient's experience of quality services. In addition to feeling under-valued and under-paid, workers are further denied the personal reward that initially attracted many to the sector — the opportunity to make a difference in the lives of other people. The inherent inflexibility of this model is further compounded by the need for providers to meet government-determined mandatory 'quality assurance' standards and training frameworks, which are enforced though monitoring, audits and complaints procedures. Being obliged to fulfil report and compliance red tape requirements under the terms of government contracts has added to large head office overheads and administration fees charged by traditional providers, which absorb a significant proportion of funding; and have both increased the cost and reduced the level of frontline service delivered locally in care recipients' homes.

A Level 4 Home Care Package offers $49,592.55 in government support per annum — a substantial sum. Yet it is common for an individual in receipt of a Level 4 package typically to receive just 10–12 hours of care per week, which is unlikely to be sufficient to care and support people assessed as having Level 4 needs and allow them to remain living in their own homes. As spelled out in monthly statements (and to the chagrin of many dissatisfied care recipients and their families), traditional provider organisations can charge between 35%–50% of funding (and sometimes more) for core administration and case management services, leaving just 65% or $32,235 available for frontline service delivery. Of the remaining funds available, service delivery is then typically charged at $45–$50 per hour during the week, the bulk of which represents the provider's margin, given that care workers are often paid $20–$27 per hour.[17] (See Figure 6)

When a Level 4 package consumer receives 10–12 hours of care per week, this means the effective cost of care is in the range of $80–$85 per hour. The deadweight loss in fewer hours of care and additional support that could be delivered from the same funding could materially improve quality of life and promote active ageing, wellness and social connection. The problem of excessive overheads is well known; a telling and typical example was documented in the federal Parliament by Andrew Wilkie MP. Citing one of the "many complaints from older Australians and their families about the ridiculous cost of home care packages", Wilkie gave the example of a "client who was effectively being charged $165 an hour ... when all the administrative expenses were included."[18]

The CDC reforms are the first, crucial step towards making the home care sector more transparent. The 'value' locked up in provider-centric models of care can now easily and conveniently be released by consumers, thanks to the introduction of CDC funding allowing new and technologically innovative players to enter the market . More efficient use of funding for service delivery not only means more hours of support for carers, but also more local jobs for care workers. (See 'Alternative Models' below.) The Uber'-style, peer-to-peer (P2P) online platforms now available to connect consumers and self-employed care workers can potentially double the amount of flexible and personalised care and support consumers receive. The introduction of choice and competition has already revealed that non-traditional, for-profit online platforms can allow consumers to access services far more efficiently and receive many more hours of care: innovative entrants into the market that are not burdened by traditional provider organisational overheads have found consumers can access 20-plus hours care per week—8 hours of additional care support (in place of paying for head office positions)— out of the same Level 4 funding package.[19]

This is consistent with the promising results of an Australian-first trial of consumer-directed aged care conducted in Western Australia. Under a pilot involving the Regional Assessment Service (RAS) and two home care providers, funding for the Home and Community Care program was converted into individualised, needs-based funding. Due to the attitudes of two forward-thinking partner organisation Avivo and MercyCare, the 103 participating clients were encouraged to exercise choice and control over the services and support they purchased. The traditional 'provider' role was transformed from fully controlling, managing and coordinating service delivery to offering information and advice about engaging their care workers directly as independent contractors. The reported (as anticipated) benefits of consumers having greater say in directing their care included savings in administration charges, higher pay for care workers, better matching of clients with workers and, in general, the ability to use funding flexibly and creatively to maximise service and support—such as by having the autonomy to purchase equipment or choose taxis over HACC transport.[20]

The financial significance for government of the innovative service delivery options now available needs underlining. Inefficient use of available government funding adversely affects the availability of packages overall. The more efficient the delivery of services, the longer recipients can remain on lower-level funding packages, and the more packages that can be funded from the available pool. But if the benefits of choice, competition and the new economy are to be realised across the sector, the CDC reforms are insufficient by themselves to achieve the desired outcome.

The broader aged care regulatory environment, including employment law, threatens to prevent innovators from helping consumers to enjoy the full benefits of the CDC reforms. For example, if governments continue to regulate quality through rigid mandatory standards and dictate how care is delivered from the top down, this could hobble the market for consumer-focused care. A focus on compliance with overarching standards and regulations threatens to limit the opportunities for real choice and competition to raise quality from the bottom up, preventing providers from discovering how best to deliver the type and mix of services that consumers want to purchase. The additional regulatory reforms suggested in this report would promote the development of "a diverse ecology of aged care providers [that] is the best guarantee of a diversity of service options for consumers", as recommended by the peak lobby organisation, the Aged Care Industry Association.[21]

Figure 6: Funding Breakdown

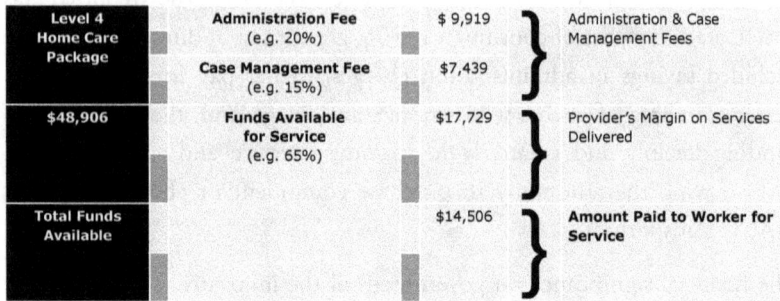

Level 4 Home Care Package	Administration Fee (e.g. 20%)	$ 9,919	Administration & Case Management Fees
	Case Management Fee (e.g. 15%)	$7,439	
$48,906	Funds Available for Service (e.g. 65%)	$17,729	Provider's Margin on Services Delivered
Total Funds Available		$14,506	Amount Paid to Worker for Service

Optimising Outcomes

Regulation

Under the historic bulk funding system, quality was regulated by requiring approved providers to comply with audited home care standards and mandatory training of care workers to enforce the development of a skilled and knowledgeable workforce.[22] Under this regulatory regime, the federal government effectively paid providers not just to deliver services, but also to manage the risks involved in caring for the elderly in their own homes. This is understandable, given the vulnerable circumstances of some care recipients. Yet this tick box, micro-management approach of requiring providers to meet a handful of easy-to-measure standards and employ qualified care workers with the requisite training certificates was no guarantee of a quality care experience for consumers. The further unintended but predictable consequence is the administrative burden and compliance costs associated with government red tape and regulation of standards, which compromised the efficiency and effectiveness of the system by increasing the cost and reducing the level of frontline services delivered locally in care recipients' homes. This also encouraged the 'institutional-style' control exercised by provider organisations over what the care workers did and when they did it—a model of care necessitated (or at least justified) on the grounds of reducing potential liability and fulfilling the providers' statutorily-imposed duty of care.

In terms of delivering quality care, it is possible both government and providers have been more focused on avoiding adverse events by meeting basic standards, and less focused on maximising outcomes and quality of life for consumers. Perpetuating the excessively risk-averse regulatory environment embedded in the culture of the sector will undermine the objectives of the CDC reforms. There is an appropriate regulatory role for government to establish minimum quality standards for providers such as police and reference checks, and insurance and basic training requirements. This is the model of regulating core safeguards favoured as best practice by the Harper competition review,[23] with the rationale being that regulation must be light, and the temptation to over-regulate must be resisted, if choice and competition are to become the major drivers of quality.

A move in this direction has been foreshadowed in the 2016 *Aged Care Roadmap* developed by the Aged Care Sector Committee at the request of the federal Government. Recognising the need for a "more proportionate regulatory framework that gives providers freedom to be innovative", the *Roadmap* envisages the creation of a single provider registration scheme, which will also encompass the development of a single set of "core standards based on their registration category and scope of practice." [24] The *Roadmap* also envisages simplified criteria and a streamlined approval process, recognising that the current application process is marred by "unnecessary red tape which creates barriers to entry", limiting the choice available to consumers by limiting the participation of new, suitable providers offering innovative models of care. A commitment to establish "a single quality framework for all aged care services" was announced by the Turnbull Government as part of the 2015–16 Budget.[25]

However, deregulation may need to go further and extend to revisiting the regulation of care workers. Requiring mandatory qualifications for care workers is an example of over-regulation, which exacerbates the well-documented workforce challenges in the sector (including the additional demand and competition for care workers created by the NDIS rollout). According to the 2015 'stocktake' prepared for the federal Department of Social Services, the aged care workforce will be required to nearly triple from 352,145 people to 827,100 people by 2050. [26]

Just because care workers have attended and completed a training course does not guarantee they will practise what they have learned, nor ensure that consumers will be guaranteed a quality experience. Quality of care is a personal experience that rests on the nature of the relationship between the consumer and the care worker, and is largely dependent on what the consumer perceives about the attitude and motivation of the care worker.

Given the 'institutionalised' style of 'rote caring' that proliferated under the old system, often involving limited personal connection between care workers and recipients, it is not surprising that consumers may prefer to hire people without industry experience and mandatory qualifications. The freedom to engage care workers without industry experience requires governments to trust consumers to make choices in their own interests, and to acknowledge that care recipients are best placed to judge the suitability of care workers based on the quality of services delivered. This would also help to address the national care worker shortage and increase the size of the care worker pool to meet the growing demand for care. [27]

Risk

Governments are likely to be wary of a minimum standards regulatory framework—and are being encouraged to do so by traditional providers who warn that the emergence of online disrupters will lead to low-paid workers delivering "second-rate" services and support.[28] However, the current array of complex and burdensome regulatory safeguards has often originated (in the words of the Productivity Commission) as an "over-reaction to specific incidents" of poor quality care or maltreatment of the elderly.[29]

In other words, regulation also serves to protect the Minister and the department when things go wrong. When media stories about incidents of poor quality aged care appear, the amount of regulation imposed can easily be cited to claim that government has done everything possible to maintain standards. Nevertheless, widely publicised failures have occurred despite the highly regulated nature of the aged care system. As Professor Ian Harper has warned, continuation of excessive and high-cost regulation will defeat the purpose of the CDC reforms by entrenching the position of incumbent providers whose business model is more or less purpose-designed to meet standards dictated under regulation, and by acting as a barrier to entry for new players that can otherwise offer consumers real choice of services based on their own assessment of quality.[30] Regulations that increase overheads will raise costs at the expense of consumers receiving less care and support, and at the expense of the wages of care workers.

Minimum standards would also address the paternalistic hangover from the old system by adopting a more dignified attitude towards the elderly and to managing risk within the system. As the Productivity Commission argued, aged care services for older people should be "delivered in ways that respect their dignity and independence."[31] The notion that providers know what's best assumes the elderly are incapable of making choices—and that they must be protected by regulation against making bad choices. This is 'institutional-style' thinking, when the point of home-based aged care is that people are capable of independent living with appropriate supports. Independence includes the capacity to live a meaningful and dignified life, which entails making decisions to improve quality of life and taking responsibility for the reasonable risks those decisions entail. Or as the Productivity Commission puts it: "people should be able to make their own life choices, even if it means they accept a higher level of risk."[32]

Allowing consumers to exercise real choice in a competitive service market will enhance, not obviate, duty of care. Yet the emphasis of the CDC reforms on consumers being best able to judge and drive quality through exercising choice is not adequately reflected in the current federal legislation. Under the new system, the role of some approved providers will change: they will no longer provide services but will continue to hold the individualised funding for consumers (see 'Unbundling' below). However, under the *Aged Care Act 1997*, approved providers remain responsible for packages and compliance with regulations, and ultimately for service provision. Revision of the Act to resolve these tensions in line with the principles, objectives and practicalities of the consumer-directed environment is needed. The legislation should clarify that, under CDC, approved provider organisations that offer fund holding services are not responsible for the quality of services independently purchased by consumers.[33]

Amendment of the Aged Care Act along these lines is especially important to avoid the current legislation being exploited by traditional providers, for example, by citing statutory obligations to fulfil standards and protect quality of care (based on internal assessments of risk and potential liability) as an excuse to deny consumers the right to choose—and remain in charge of delivering—the entire package. Terminological change is needed to reflect the CDC realities within the sector. The term 'approved provider' is redundant and reflects the norms of the old bulk-funded system. The *Aged Care Roadmap* suggests that the term 'registered provider' or 'recognised provider' will gain official currency, and notes the need for reconsideration of provider responsibilities and new compliance pathways and monitoring of standards consistent with the changed role of providers in a consumer-driven system.[34]

While the proposed new terminology will somewhat reflect the change of status under the CDC system, the use of 'provider' still implies that organisations whose exclusive and primary functions may now be limited to fund holding are in fact providers of services. Establishing new and accurate terminology—'Registered CDC Fund-Holder' comes to mind—will help foster consumer awareness of individualised funding and the right to choose.

Independent Contractors

A core or minimum standards regulatory framework will also help break down workplace rigidities and amplify the flexibility and responsiveness of consumer-directed care. An expanded care workforce would not necessarily need to be employed and rostered by provider organisations, but could be self-employed—literally cutting out middle management in service delivery– and be hired as independent contractors by empowered consumers. The rigid model of 'rote care by roster' would become a thing of the past, starting with consumers being free to access services when they want and need them, such as in the evening and on the weekend.

Independent contracting would make employment as a care worker more desirable and rewarding by addressing the hierarchical structures and low pay and low status that deter people from pursuing a career in the sector. Allowing consumers to contract directly with their care workers, and be able to set and negotiate agreed fees—which is an inherently more professional, client-based employment relationship—would apply to aged care the same principles of choice and contestability that consumers are familiar with in other human services sectors, including GP services, allied healthcare and dental care. Compensation for self-employment and the loss of traditional employee benefits includes not only much greater work flexibility but also the opportunity for workers to invest in their own knowledge and skills, develop niche specialised services, and build their own businesses as independent care contractors. [35]

The introduction of individualised funding for disability services under the NDIS has increased demand for self-employed support and care workers.[36] This is consistent with the world-wide trend towards self-employment across a range of industries, as noted by the 2015 Committee for the Economic Development (CEDA) report, Australia's Future Workforce.[37] Independent contracting of home care workers is possible under the CDC system, and due to the emergence of alternative, non-traditional online platforms that allow care workers to be engaged independently by multiple (demanding) consumers to provide personalised services. Because these online platforms—as noted above—release funding tied up in the excessive administration charges of traditional providers, they allow care workers to be paid more to deliver more care, while giving care and support workers the opportunity to take responsibility for the quality of care by responding to consumer need and developing the personal relationship and connection with care recipients in ways that make a substantial difference to quality of life.

To nurture the growth of the new economy in home care services, government action is needed concerning workplace legislation. Potential confusion arises under current employment laws as to whether the consumer is employing or contracting the care worker. To enable real choice, consumers need clarity around employing and contracting workers for personal services and domestic services so that local consumers and care workers can negotiate flexible and mutually beneficial arrangements.[38] A consumer who directly engages a care worker—when the intent of both parties is a flexible contracting arrangement—could also potentially be interpreted under existing laws to be creating an employment relationship subject to existing industry award conditions—a line of argument that could be advanced by unions (and some traditional providers intent on preserving control over both fund holding and service delivery) in proceedings before the Fair Work Commission. This is a common problem across disruptive industries, and determining the status of workers as either an employee or independent contractor is being worked out on a case by case basis.[39] One way to provide certainty for consumers and care workers would be for independent contracting for home care services to be carved out from existing laws and extended legislative relief from sham contracting provisions.[40]

Unbundling

The success of the CDC system relies on changing the cultural and social assumptions about the elderly that have surrounded aged care services. Many elderly people have the capacity to control their own lives by making choices about their care and support services based on self-assessed needs and preferences. Some elderly consumers will need to make these choices in consultation with family and advocates. And some (including those with dementia and other cognitive defects or limited language skills) may need to have their choices guided and have their care case-managed by providers, ideally in concert with independent advocates or other proxy decision makers.[41] However, the current situation, where all consumers are effectively denied choice by having their care case-managed by traditional providers, is unnecessary and inconsistent with the goal of consumer-directed care.

Traditional providers bundle case management into their one-size-fits-all care package, along with fund holding, administration, care coordination, advocacy and service delivery. A full package may be appropriate for some consumers, including perhaps the most vulnerable elderly. However, vulnerable and disadvantaged people should still have access to impartial advice to help guide their choices as recommended by the Harper Review.[42] If consumers are to exercise real choice, unbundling of traditional packages is required to enable people to pick and choose the mix of services that is right for them. Unbundling could proceed through the emergence of specialised organisations offering different parts of the bundle and components of care that can each be purchased discretely. Advocacy services are currently offered free of charge through the My Aged Care website.[43] However, to ensure consumers are properly informed about their care needs, specialist organisations could emerge offering independent advocacy and impartial, easy-to-understand advice and case management without offering services.[44]

Unbundling could involve consumers receiving a personalised care plan, while retaining the freedom to purchase services independently. This could include choosing an individual independent contractor care worker ahead of an approved provider, whose role in delivering unbundled packages would change to offering only to host and administer the funding at the direction of consumers. Unbundling makes possible real choice of services and service providers by enabling consumers to access the innovative technological solutions that are now available—the P2P online platforms that offer real-time brokerage services for consumers without the excessive overheads of traditional bundled care packages.

Alternative Models

P2P Platforms

Despite the advent of consumer-directed care, many traditional provider organisations fear the consequences for their businesses of transparent competition on cost and quality of services. Some, in defence of their generous margins, are therefore keen to limit consumers' right to exercise choice, denying them the opportunity to seek better outcomes. This may succeed in part due to many care recipients being unaware of their rights under the new system—an information gap government could remedy through an appropriate education and awareness campaign.

However, there are also reports of providers having scrambled—ahead of the introduction of full portability on 27 February—to introduce barriers to choice in the form of charging exit fees for consumers wishing to choose a different service provider.[45] This is on top of other concerns about "the high barriers to change including the time it may take [up to 10 weeks] to transfer unspent home care amounts."[46] Imposing large switching costs creates an unlevel playing field contrary to the spirit and intent of the CDC reforms.[47]

The federal government has allowed providers to charge exit amounts (and retrospectively include such charges in home care agreements) on the questionable grounds of allowing them to "recover administrative costs associated with determining and making payment of unspent home care amounts."[48] Nevertheless, the government should signal its strong disapproval of the charging of hefty exit fees by traditional providers keen to lock consumers into existing contracts. To encourage providers to cease this practice, it may be sufficient for the government to foreshadow the application of Australian consumer law, which according to the Combined Pensioners and Superannuants Association "states that a person has the right to cancel a service without incurring fees if that service was...unfit for the purpose you asked for".[49]

For real choice to occur, consumers also need to be aware of the innovative options that are now available alongside traditional providers. Across a variety of sectors of the economy—from taxis and travel to retail, music and education—disruptive technology is empowering consumers, connecting people in new transparent and efficient markets, and raising the quality and lowering the cost of services. The rise of a tech-enabled new economy in aged care is the solution that can deliver real choice for increasing numbers of elderly consumers needing care and support to live independently in their own homes cared for by an increasingly large number of care workers required to provide care and support locally.

These innovative solutions are already operating today. Consumer-directed funding has enabled new providers to enter the Australian aged care (and disability support) sector offering online P2P marketplaces for care and support services. P2P organisations support the right to choose by enabling access to an online platform—a website or app—which allows care recipients (or their family members, advocates or case managers) quickly and conveniently to purchase the kind of services desired. Consumer-focused P2P platforms expand the available choices by allowing consumers to access the services of competing provider organisations or individual care workers (operating as independent contractors).

P2P organisations can afford to charge much lower administrative fees—in the vicinity of 15% of the cost of care—with care workers paying a fee of 10% of their hourly agreed rate and consumers a 5% fee on top of the agreed rate. Lower overheads compared to traditional providers release additional funding to allow consumers to purchase more services—approximately 70% more care and support per week out of a CDC package as noted above—and improve care worker remuneration to help draw workers to the industry. This is especially the case in regional, rural and remote regions with greatest need and limited access to services: low-cost online platforms connect local consumers and care workers in these areas where traditional high-cost providers cannot afford to operate—creating local jobs in local communities instead of head office middle management positions. P2P marketplaces can therefore help solve workforce challenges and drive job creation in both urban and rural locations by offering more flexible and attractive opportunities for care workers operating as independent contractors.[50]

P2P market places also permit aged care provision to occur in a minimum standards regulatory framework, and are the key to resolving the conflict between the vision of a flexible consumer-driven, independent contractor-based system, and the existing regulation of home care standards. P2P organisations ensure care workers meet basic checks, policies and procedures but quality would be community-regulated. P2P market places ensure accountability through transparent feedback from consumers on their experience—by the ratings and comments made on provider sites that inform the choices of other consumers. Choice and competition become the ultimate safeguard of standards, since care workers who fail to provide high quality care and satisfy customers' needs and expectations will not be able to function on the platform—as is the case in any industry subject to disruptive technology.

Public Information Campaign

Ensuring consumers can exercise real choice also depends, in the first instance, on fostering greater awareness of the fact that consumers now have the right to choose. As analysts of the sector have rightly warned, "consumers might not be able to find the right aged care provider if their choices are limited by lack of information."[51] According to a survey by researchers at the University of SA, University of Adelaide and Torrens University: "Only 11 per cent of respondents to our survey had heard of CDC, and only 22 per cent of those who were aware of CDC (2 per cent of the population of older people) had a sound understanding of its entirety."[52]

A government-funded public information campaign is needed to complement and complete the final stage of the CDC rollout—full portability from 27 February, 2017. This would be similar to the public education campaign conducted by the NSW Government to inform people with a disability about the NDIS.[53]

Education for consumers about the CDC changes should include information about how to switch providers, and personal stories of consumers making choices and achieving better outcomes by switching (as is the case with the NSW NDIS campaign). It should also include information about individualised budgets and provider charges, and about accessing impartial and independent advice.

The biggest service a government-funded public information campaign might render would be to challenge the established culture of the sector regarding the key issues of choice and risk. Education of providers and consumers alike is needed around the concept of duty of care—which should be redefined to a more reasonable and balanced definition that encompasses people's right to choose, as opposed to providers inhibiting choice on the basis that they have to manage risk.

Fostering greater awareness of innovative online options should also be a key objective, regardless of the objections of traditional providers whose interests are threatened by greater choice and transparency. Fear of upsetting key stakeholders with vested interests (and ready access to media prepared to run "embarrassing" anti-private sector, pro-'charity' stories) may explain why the federal government is running relatively quietly on the full introduction of the CDC system—at the expense of leaving consumers in the dark about the new private sector care options now available, and thereby jeopardising the success of the key reforms. Consumers have a right to be informed about the full range of government-funded services available if they are to exercise real choice, and should not be denied knowledge of the innovative models that can deliver better value and quality.

Reforms Must Go Far Enough to Achieve Real Choice

The shift to the consumer-directed aged care system presents an important opportunity to showcase the benefits of market-based reforms to sceptical and change-averse members of the public. However, optimising the outcomes achieved for consumers, care workers and taxpayers depends on government willingness to pursue additional regulatory reforms in order to maximise the provision, value and quality of aged care services at minimal additional cost.

Legislative clarification of providers' role and duty of care and clarification of employment laws to confirm the status of independent contractor care workers are required to facilitate real consumer choice and competition. Enabling innovative and efficient online platforms to challenge the dominance of traditional providers will help to connect consumers directly with the kind of care they want, when they want it, from the care worker they want to deliver those services. By improving the quality of services received, a competitive and transparent market for aged care will improve the quality of life enjoyed by many ageing Australians.

The federal government's role as market steward in nurturing the success of consumer-directed care should include ensuring consumers do not face significant switching costs by foreshadowing the application of Australian consumer law to the charging of hefty exit fees. This is indicative of the wider educative role the federal government should play to maximise awareness of the new CDC system through a public information campaign that makes consumers aware of their right to choose and the choices available including innovative online P2P market places. Encouraging consumers to exercise greater choice would be money well spent, given the potential benefits for care recipients accessing more support and services, for care workers afforded new employment opportunities in local communities, and for taxpayers funding more efficient and financially sustainable home care packages.

Real consumer choice means diversity of provision. P2P platforms allow individual consumers and individual workers (independent contractors) to strike highly personalised and mutually beneficial agreements without the added cost of traditional providers in the middle. Workers who value independence and control over their employment, who are motivated by making a difference to the quality of lives of their elderly clients in a commercially accountable environment, will be attracted to the sector by the new employment opportunities created by disruptive technology. The flexibility, fulfilment and superior financial rewards on offer will help solve the workforce challenges facing the sector, especially in non-metropolitan Australia where service shortages are chronic.

P2P care workers will deliver the kind of care consumers want to receive, not the kind of care providers want to deliver. The demanding and informed baby boomer demographic that will be exercising their right to choose in coming decades will not accept the status quo of 'institutionalised' care in their own home, particularly when many will be contributing to the means-tested cost of their care. Traditional provider models (and the corresponding regulatory framework), whether those organisations like it or not, are out of date and must adapt and innovate—or perish. This reality is already dawning on established service providers in the disability services sector in the wake of the rollout of the $22 billion NDIS, which has finally empowered consumers dissatisfied with traditional providers to take their business to the "number of new, more innovative, cost-efficient and consumer-responsive startups, multinational for-profits, and sole-traders entering this market."[54]

Aged care services, too, must join the modern world and the new economy, and continuing reforms must go as far as necessary to achieve the optimal, desired outcomes. Further action by government to nurture the aged care market is needed to give consumers real choice and control over the services they want to receive. The regulatory barriers that will otherwise restrict consumer choice and limit genuine competition among traditional providers and innovators must be removed to give ageing Australians greater access to efficient and effective consumer-focused aged care services.

Endnotes

1   Harper, I. et al., Competition Policy Review, the Commonwealth of Australia, 2015.

2   Sammut, Thomas, Seaton, Medi-Vation: Health Innovation Communities for Medicare Payment and Service Reform Research Report 21, (Sydney: The Centre for Independent Studies, 2016).

3   http://www.afr.com/technology/carers-marketplace-better-caring-raises-3-million-from-ellerston-ventures-20161018-gs4n1o

4   2015 Intergenerational Report Australia in 2055, (Canberra: Commonwealth of Australia, 2015).

5   http://www.smh.com.au/business/aged-care-funding-cuts-set-to-drive-industry-consolidation-20160504-gom3m5.html

6   Deloitte Access Economics Aged Care Guild, Australia's Aged Care Sector: Economic Contribution and Future Directions, 12

7   Living Longer. Living Better. Aged Care Reform Package, April 2012, 3

8   The Treasury, Nick Sherry, Assistant Treasurer, joint media release with the Hon Justine Elliot MP Minister for Ageing: Productivity Commission Inquiry into Aged Care, No. 068.

9   Henry, K. et al., Australia's Future Tax System: Report to the Treasurer, The Treasury, 2009.

10 Drape, J., FED: Aged care sector pleased with Henry's nod to less regulation, AAP General News Wire, 03 May 2010.

11 Productivity Commission, Caring for Older Australians, (Canberra: 2011).

12 Lunn, S., Julia Gillard's bid to avert crisis in Aged Care, The Australian, 21 April 2012.

13 Living Longer. Living Better. Aged Care Reform Package, 3-4.

14 Deloitte Access Economics Aged Care Guild, Australia's Aged Care Sector: Economic Contribution and Future Directions, 2.

15 T.H. Kewley, Social Services in Australia, 5-19.

16 https://cipher.org.au/why-consumer-directed-aged-care-is-good-policy/

17 Better Caring Pty Limited—Submission to Aged Care Legislated Review, 3; Better Caring PTY Limited Submission, Productivity Commission Inquiry into Human Services, 7; Better Caring PTY Limited Submission, Senate Standing Committee on Community Affairs Inquiry on The Future of Australia's aged care sector workforce, 7.

18 Hansard, 14 September 2016.

19 Better Caring PTY Limited Submission, Productivity Commission Inquiry into Human Services, 13-14

20 'Providers demonstrate benefits of CDC in home support: trial', Community Care Review, 1 December 2016.

21 Aged Care Industry Association, Submission to Aged Care Legislated Review, 5.

22 ttps://agedcare.health.gov.au/sites/g/files/net1426/f/documents/09_2014/community_care_standard_guidelines2.pdf

23 Harper, 37.

24 Aged Care Sector Committee, Aged Care Roadmap,(Canberra: 2016) 3.

25 Aged Care Roadmap, 10, 13.

26 https://agedcare.health.gov.au/stocktake-and-analysis-of-commonwealth-funded-aged-care-workforce-activities-final-report

27 Better Caring PTY Limited Submission, Senate Standing Committee on Community Affairs Inquiry on the Future of Australia's aged care sector workforce, 4.

28 http://cdn5.australianageingagenda.com.au/wp-content/uploads/2016/05/Keeping-the-mission-in-the-market.pdf

29 Productivity Commission, Caring for Older Australians, xlii.

30 'Competition will increase responsiveness of community care: Harper', Community Care Review, 25 February, 2016.

31 Productivity Commission, Caring for Older Australians, xix.

32 Productivity Commission, Caring for Older Australians, xxiii.

33 Better Caring Pty Limited—Submission to Aged Care Legislated Review, 6.

34 Aged Care Roadmap, 3, 10.

35 http://www.australianageingagenda.com.au/2016/06/01/embracing-new-models-key-aged-cares-future/

36 http://theconversation.com/new-risks-for-disability-care-workers-under-the-ndis-63812

37 Ken Phillips, 'Your future employer—yourself', CEDA, Australia's Future Workforce, (CEDA, 2015), 3.3.

38 Better Caring PTY Limited Submission, Productivity Commission Inquiry into Human Services, 17.

39 http://theconversation.com/workers-are-taking-on-more-risk-in-the-gig-economy-61797

40 Better Caring Pty Limited—Submission to Aged Care Legislated Review, 10.

41 Productivity Commission, Caring for Older Australians, XL.

42 Harper, Competition Policy Review, 44.

43 http://www.myagedcare.gov.au/quality-and-complaints/advocacy-services

44 Better Caring PTY Limited Submission, Productivity Commission Inquiry into Human Services, 12.

45 Better Caring Pty Limited—Submission to Aged Care Legislated Review, 7.

46 http://www.afr.com/personal-finance/home-care-changes-beware-potential-rorts-20170110-gtotfu#ixzz4ZAPGtLY4

47 See Harper, Competition Policy Review, 36.

48 https://agedcare.health.gov.au/programs/home-care/overview-of-exit-amounts

49 http://www.cpsa.org.au/aged-care/1499-home-care-exit-fees-by-stealth

50 Better Caring Pty Limited—Submission to Aged Care Legislated Review, 8.

51 Rhonda Lynette-Smith and Ian Martin McDonald, More competition may not be the answer to reforming t the aged care system', The Conversation, 27 May 2016.

52 The University of South Australia; The University of Adelaide; and Torrens University Australia Submission, Aged Care Legislated Review, 6.

53 http://www.smh.com.au/national/how-siobahn-daley-became-the-public-face-of-the-ndis-20161104-gsi2c1.html

54 'How the disability sector is being uberised', Australian Financial Review, 6 October 2016.

Chapter 5

Improving Palliative Care
for Older Australians*

Jessica Borbasi

Introduction: Why Palliative Care Matters

The Australian health system is struggling to deliver high quality healthcare for all Australians in an affordable way, in the face of well-known and mounting challenges. The rising cost of health — which already consumes 10% of GDP annually — is being largely driven by the impact of the ageing of the population on demand for health services. Paradoxically, these challenges have arisen due to how successful modern medicine has been in prolonging average lifespans over the past 60 years.

Health systems such as Australia's that operate around the model of 'treat and cure' excel at delivering effective short-term treatment for short-term acute illnesses. But ageing Australians ultimately develop incurable chronic conditions. This incongruence — between the needs of the community and the type of medicine supplied — highlights how the health system is struggling to deal with the number one health challenge facing the nation: the effective treatment and management of the rising burden of chronic disease in the twenty-first century.[1]

The consequences of keeping more people with chronic disease alive for longer, with a system not fit for this purpose, has not gone unnoticed. "The patient experience of care receives little focus as a goal of the system. Notwithstanding the massive burden of chronic illness, its prevention and

---

* Originally published as Life Before Death: Improving Palliative Care for Older Australians, Research Report 34, (Sydney: The Centre for Independent Studies, 2017).

proper management is still in its infancy."[2] The Harper competition and policy review suggested that "without fundamental change to the health and aged care systems, the ageing of Australia's population will mean a future of greater government-managed care and increased rationing of health services."

Chronic disease sufferers need to receive integrated or coordinated, person-centred care that will allow them access to all necessary multidisciplinary care in the lowest cost setting, and prevent inefficiencies such as avoidable hospital admissions. Palliative care upholds these characteristics and has been identified as a priority area for reform. The Productivity Commission's 2016 review of Australia's human services suggested there be an increase in user choice about the setting, timing and availability of care in light of the fact that currently there is substantial variation in the quality of palliative care services across Australia.[3]

The most recent Inquiry Report similarly argued that "the system primarily responds to patient crisis. In areas where patient choice is critical—an exemplar being end-of-life care—many people are disempowered because they do not get adequate access to end-of-life care at home, but are instead treated in a hospital setting." The NSW Auditor similarly concluded that "NSW Health has a limited understanding of the quantity and quality of palliative care services across the state, and at a district level planning is ad hoc and accountability for performance is unclear."[4]

The reality is that most Australians don't receive palliative care in approaching death, and too many elderly Australians don't even live well before they die. As this chapter shows, some estimates are that as many as 130,000 Australians should have received palliative care last year, but approximately only 14,300 did. Other estimates are that at least 20% of hospital patients would benefit from palliative care, but the majority who would benefit do not receive palliative care services.

Due to more accurate estimates of cancer mortality, and the clinical culture and funding of oncology services, patients dying from cancer are more likely (up to eight times more likely according to some estimates) to receive palliative care. However, the preferential provision for patients suffering from cancer is the exception to the rule. Access to palliative care in Australia is limited or non-existent for the majority of Australians who do not die from cancer but from 'diseases of ageing' each year, and is suboptimal amongst particular groups—including those with non-malignant disease, as well as those in hospital and residential aged care facilities. Patchy provision of palliative care, and inadequate access based on location, diagnosis, background, and doctor, is due to a range of historical cultural and institutional barriers within the health system, the medical profession, and in the community and across government, including persistent workforce and funding challenges.

Old age and death are humbling phenomena that make equals of us all. Yet for too many older Australians, the experience lacks the autonomy, dignity, and compassion that palliative care can provide. As the population grows to older ages with increasing frailty, comorbidities and expectations the need for more palliative care increases. Most older Australians have multiple chronic diseases and rely heavily on the health system.

The changing nature of disease and death—to become the result of an interplay of chronic disease, frailty and medicine — is largely evidenced by the increasing longevity we are witnessing in contemporary Australia among the baby boomer generation and beyond. The typical experience of death today is very different to decades ago when heart disease or stroke killed quickly at younger ages; with the majority of Australians now dying at very old ages from *chronic* diseases. The medical revolution of recent decades has yielded enormous successes in curative medicine in an array of disease sub-specialities that have prolonged life spans and contributed significantly to the ageing of the population.

The projected 4 million Australians aged 65 and older in 2021 will—based on current trends—have on average 4 diagnosed chronic diseases and visit the GP roughly 10 times a year; using twice as many health resources as the younger Australian. Today's 65-year-old can expect to live to 87 years of age. For the average 65-year-old, this means another 22 years at least of dependency on their GP and eventually dependency on family, friends, volunteers, hospitals, ambulances and residential aged care facilities.

Whilst medicine is to be commended for providing such unprecedented longevity, the lived experience of these conditions is that they have a high symptom burden with frequent exacerbations, often requiring hospitalisation—and eventually cause a death that is unpredicted, prolonged and most often ill-managed and expensive. Not surprisingly, most Australians die in hospital and without palliative care. In the absence of palliative care, patients are highly likely to receive disjointed, inflexible, reactionary, and non-holistic care, which will be determined by what doctors decide they can do to prolong life, rather than according to what patients and their families value in life. In many cases, the over-medicalisation—and the depersonalisation and dehumanisation—of death will involve multiple and often lengthy hospital admissions, intensive 'curative' interventions, with an overall lack of acknowledgement of impending death.

Ironically, therefore, inadequate provision of palliative care is attributable to the inappropriate application of the 'treat, cure, repeat' model of *acute* health care that has successfully extended life, but which is not fit for purpose to deal with the new realities of modern death and dying at increasingly older ages. To date, the health system has been largely unable to adapt from its curative reactionary model of care to the holistic supportive care of these conditions. The barriers to greater access to palliative care are steeped in policy limitations, funding arrangements (related to the structure of Medicare), workforce issues, and cultural obstacles within both the medical profession and the wider Australian community.

The structural problems of the health system are driven by outdated funding incentives borne of a time when chronic disease wasn't the most important health issue and contribute to the inherent rigidity of the health system. Myths and horror stories about death in the Australian health system has fostered the belief that 'natural' death, with all the apparently inevitable interventions and complications, represents the antithesis of a dignified ending. Not surprisingly, these assumptions are of great concern to increasing numbers of dependent and vulnerable older Australians, who want a much better experience of life and death.

This is also fostering interest and support for more radical end-of-life options. What is missing in this debate is an appreciation of the role of palliative care, and the need to address the rigidities in the health system that currently limit the availability of palliative services. Greater access to palliative care provides the best answer—ethically and financially—for improving the way elderly Australians experience life before death as well as death itself.

The Harper review specifically suggested that the ageing population—beyond aged care arrangements—will demand "new competitive and innovative services to meet a widening array of needs and preferences."[5] The Productivity Commission concluded that "fundamental change must revolve around the greater adoption of market economy ideals including a focus on consumer, rather than producer."

What is palliative care and how can it make life better?

Palliative care is often misunderstood as purely end-of-life care. However, palliative care is not just about improving the experience of the terminal phase of life or 'dying well'. In fact, palliative care—properly defined—is a form of chronic disease management that can help address the wider challenges facing the health system. Expanding access to palliative care services in Australia would ensure that patients with incurable chronic conditions receive evidence-based, person-centred and cost-effective care—not only in the terminal stage, but earlier—to improve the quality of their lives in the period well before death.

Palliative medicine is a branch of medicine that is concerned with symptomatology and the daily experience of life as driven by patient values. Palliative care offers quality care directed by patient values that aims to ensure life before death is based on what patients and their families want and need. Palliative care upholds the values of autonomy and individuality by creating a partnership with patients. It directs care away from being curative and reactionary to being holistic and supportive by collaborating with patients, families and carers in addressing spiritual and psychosocial as well as physical concerns. It provides effective pain and symptom management, improved quality of life, improved mood, and greater patient and family satisfaction with care.[6]

Palliative care — properly defined — prevents and relieves the suffering of patients associated with chronic or incurable illness through early identification, comprehensive assessment and treatment of pain and other psychosocial or spiritual needs. Palliative care involves the delivery of coordinated, person-centred 'team care' to ensure that patients are empowered and receive the care they want and need. Palliative care offers support for patients to live as actively as possible until death, by using an interdisciplinary team approach that acknowledges dying as a normal process, but affirms life. A wealth of Australian and international evidence shows palliative care improves quality of life for both patients — by managing symptoms, including pain — and their families, by supporting patients to be as active as possible prior to death. There is extensive evidence demonstrating that palliative care is also cost effective in preventing hospitalisations, emergency transfers and unwarranted medical intervention in hospitals.

The WHO definition of palliative care is widely used in Australia:

> An approach that improves the quality of life of patients and their families facing the problem associated with life-threatening illness, through the prevention and relief of suffering by means of early identification and impeccable assessment and treatment of pain and other problems, physical, psychosocial and spiritual.[7]

Interestingly, the United States (US) health system has taken an even broader definition. In the US, palliative care extends into a patient's life even when death is not expected. That is, the patients do not have a terminal condition but rather have multiple chronic conditions with an increasing symptom burden — much like Australia's ageing population. The US palliative care team advocates for patients by communicating patient wishes with their treating specialists.[8]

Arguably, the definition of palliative care within Australia — while holistic — is not as applicable across a patient's lifespan as in the US, where palliative care is considered a solution to the changing demographic and health of the population.[9] There is significant danger in Australia of palliative care being reduced to care provided at the terminal phase — underestimating the benefits for patients and their families in their lives before death.[10]

Most patients who receive palliative care are not in pain when they die, most patients do not request to hasten death, and most patients are not fearful.[11] The rare but prevalent[12] desire to hasten death has a multifactorial aetiology and is mostly seen as a severe emotional response[13] to an overwhelming situation.[14] In Australia, less than 1% of patients receiving inpatient palliative care had a sustained request to hasten their death.[15]

All clinicians should be able to provide palliative care and end-of-life care and refer to palliative medicine specialists for more complex and difficult cases. However, the reality is many clinicians cannot and do not provide it, despite the increasing need for access to palliative services in an ageing Australia.

Ageing Australia—caring for the baby boomers and beyond

The average Australian woman who is currently 65 years of age can expect to live to 87 years and the average current 85-year-old now will live to 92.[17] The life expectancy at birth is currently 91 years for men and 93 years for women.[18] This is projected to increase to 95 years for men and 96 years for women by 2054.[19] Predictions are that the number of centenarians in 2034 will be 15,700, compared to 4,600 in 2014.[20]

The ageing Australian population is partly a product of continued low fertility rates,[21] combined with the ageing of the baby boomer generation — the large cohort of the population born between 1946 and 1964 — and compounded by the impact of improvements in medicine (including public health) that have increased longevity and reduced death rates. The baby boomers' effect on the age structure of the population will peak in 2021. However, the nation will continue to experience unprecedented population ageing as the proportion of older people increases well beyond the life spans of the baby boomer generation.[22]

In 2021, 17.6% of Australians (4 million people) — the peak of the ageing Baby Boomers — will be aged 65 years and over, compared to 1997's 12% of the population (2.2 million). By 2051, of the total expected population of 26 million, 24% or 6.3 million Australians will be aged 65 and over.[23] The number of 'very old' Australians — aged 85 and over — is also forecast to rise from 2% of the population to 5% by 2061.[24] Median population age is another measure of population ageing. Historically a population is considered old if its median age is over 30.[25] The median age of Australia in 2016 was 37; in 2021, it is forecast to be 41, and rise to 46 in 2051.[26]

The increased longevity of the population that is attributable to improvements in health, and to the changing nature of disease, is in turn changing the way people die. The median age at death has increased to 78.9 for men and 85 for women across Australia.[27] It is as high as 80.1 for men and 85.9 for women in South Australia. The majority of deaths occur among those aged 65 or over. The age-standardised death rate in Australia has actually fallen throughout the twentieth century, contributing to longevity.[28] Today it is steady at around 5.5 per 1000 population. However, a greater number of older people means an increase in the crude number of deaths per year; in 2015 there were 159,052 deaths. This is expected to increase to up to 352,100 by 2061 and beyond.[29] The leading cause of death for older Australians has been cardiovascular or heart disease for most of the twentieth century; however, this is likely to be overtaken by dementia — a degenerative disease inextricably linked to ageing.[30]

The changing experience of health, ageing, illness and death for older Australians

That more Australians will eventually die from a 'disease of ageing' is one example of how longevity has changed the experience of death. Dementia, not even appropriately recognised or recorded prior to 1979 when the death rate was 2.35 per 100,000 population, is now the second leading cause of death.[31]

Greater longevity has fortunately meant in general a greater number of years lived without disability; and this is despite people living with several chronic health issues, as these are managed with modern medicine.

This increased period of active ageing, with chronic disease, is largely attributable to public health, medical sub specialisation and treatment. There are currently 85 specialist titles recognised by the Medical Board of Australia, which doesn't include sub specialisation e.g. interventional cardiologist or subsubspecialisation e.g. advanced heart failure and transplant cardiology.[32] In the 1970s, there were 20 medical specialties. Specialisation has allowed us to treat diseases so well that the way they impact life, and eventually cause death, has changed. It is an irony that the experience of death (from chronic disease) for many Australians has changed for the worse, despite living longer. Chronic diseases are incurable, co-exist, persist and contribute to a gradual deterioration of health, symptom burden, loss of independence and ultimately, at increasingly greater ages, death.[33]

Causes of death over the last century tell the story of how Australians have a changed experience of health and death. Circulatory diseases—including cerebrovascular disease (mainly stroke) and ischemic heart disease—experienced a great rise as the dominant cause of death during the twentieth century. However, improved treatments meant the death rates fell; for example from 1,020 male deaths per 100,000 in 1968 to 319 per 100,000 in 2000. Cardiovascular disease still remains the leading cause of death, however the age at which death occurs has changed so that the cumulative number of deaths from circulatory disease began to peak by the age of 45 in 1970, but by the year 2000 it was 85.[34]

Death rates from respiratory diseases, including pneumonia, influenza and chronic obstructive pulmonary disease (COPD), also peaked and then fell collectively over the century. Within the group, COPD has increased relative to pneumonia, which has declined dramatically as a cause of death. Death rates from infectious diseases were around 7 deaths per 100,000 population for females in 2000—a far cry from 230 per 100,000 in 1907. Tuberculosis was the leading cause of death in women in 1907. Now it is ischemic heart disease, cerebrovascular disease, other heart disease and dementia. However, in the very old age group—those over 85—death from septicaemia has increased since the 1980s, probably because more people are reaching this age and we have increasing antibiotics resistance.[35]

Death rates from cancer at the beginning of the twentieth century were initially half that of circulatory disease. The all cancer death rate then peaked for men in 1980 at 290 deaths per 100,000 population; it has since declined to 234.4 per 100,000 in 2003. Among this category, deaths from lung cancer have continued to rise as a hangover from the previous popularity of smoking. Smoking cessation is also attributable to the reduced death rates from ischemic heart disease, and other cancers over the course of the twentieth century. (Figure 7)

Figure 7: Age-standardised death rates, by broad cause of death, 1907-2014

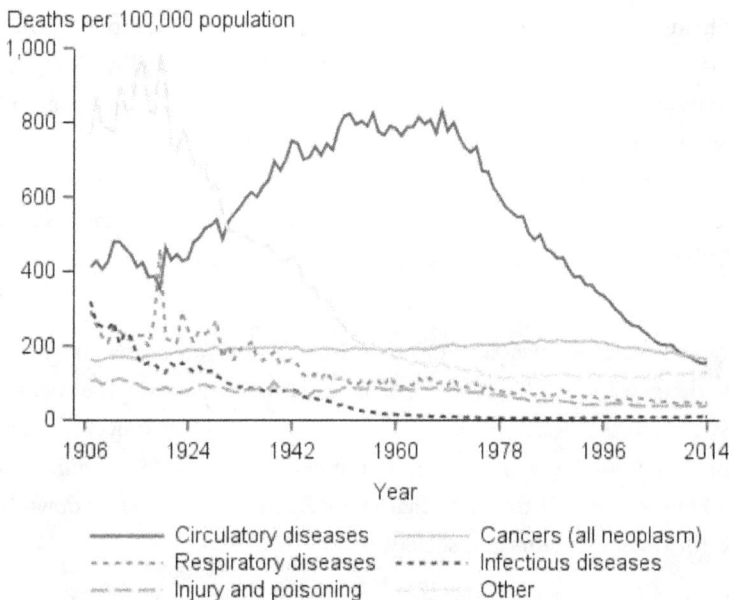

Source: AIHW GRIM books (Data tables)

The increase in longevity and rise in the chronic disease burden due to improved treatments is reflected in the typical Australian over 65 having four chronic diseases and visiting the GP roughly 10 times a year—using twice as many health resources as the average Australian.[36] Older people are the largest per capita consumers of medications. GPs prescribe around 120 medications per 100 encounters with those aged over 65[37] who are estimated to account for two thirds of prescriptions filled under the PBS and roughly half the PBS's total expenditure—which is projected to reach over 15 billion dollars by 2023.[38] The amount of polypharmacy, as defined by five or more medications, is increasing proportional to the ageing population and increasing comorbidity of chronic diseases.[39]

Due to medical intervention—that of specialists, GPs and medications—cancer, stroke, ischemic heart disease and respiratory disease have become chronic conditions. Patients need significant support to maintain 'health' until death. It is testament to our health system that most older Australians, rate their health as 'good', confirming the success of medicine in managing chronic diseases and delaying disability.[40] Women aged 65 can expect to live another 9.5 years free of disability, 6.7 years with a disability but no severe or profound core activity limitation, and 5.8 years with a severe core activity limitation such as always needing assistance with either self-care, mobilising, or communication (8.7, 6.7, and 3.7 years for men, respectively). This corresponds to around 86% of Australians aged over 85 requiring some form of assistance compared to 32% of those aged 65–74 years.[41]

Decline and dependence is inevitable, but is now occurring at greater ages with increasing frailty. Older Australians are relying on the medical profession and the health system to keep them well—but prevention and treatment can only do so much before the deterioration into disability and death. However, it is at this time that many Australians will be let down by the health system, doctors and society.

The pattern of life in the months before death is usually evidenced by ongoing exacerbations, readmissions and interventions, until an unexpected death in hospital. In 2013–2014 and 2015–2016, almost 50% of Australians died in hospital. The remaining 50% of Australians likely die in RACFs, or at home, however there is a lack of data clearly demonstrating where Australians die.

A study of over 7000 Australian decedents who died from cancer and non-cancer causes found that in the last six months of life, the mean number of hospitalisations per person was 3.1, and these increased—together with emergency department presentations—in the last month of life. The average total cost of health care per decedent in the last six months of life was AUD $30,001 in the cohort who died from cancer and $26,131 in the non-cancer comparison cohort. The majority in both cohorts died in hospital.[42]

Elderly patients with chronic diseases experiencing back-to-back readmissions are rarely given the opportunity to receive care based on their values and choices; such as staying at home rather than living longer with curative intent. Instead, many end up dying suddenly in an emergency department, or after lingering for days, weeks or months in a hospital ward or intensive care bed—to the distress of both the patient and their family.

These experiences[43] demonstrate how the current health system is not fit for purpose in managing older Australians with chronic disease. The doctor-directed model of treatment seems aimed at prolonging life irrespective of costs. Often, a variety of specialists across multiple settings deliver reactionary care in response to specific clinical indications, which are delivered through a prism of 'treat and cure', rather than holistic goal-orientated care that is centred around the needs of the 'whole patient'.

For example, for most Australians quality of life means growing old at home.[44] Already Australians are facing shortages of aged care places, in-home assistance, palliative care and family support. Staying at home will become even more difficult to ensure as a smaller proportion of the population is available to provide and pay for aged care services in an ageing Australia. The way we care for elderly Australians currently drains services that are already under strain (See Box 5).

Box 5: Services are already under strain

- In 2015 there were already an estimated 2.86 million people—mostly women aged 55-65 years—providing informal care in Australia. They provided roughly 1.9 billion hours worth of care, the replacement value of which is estimated to be $60.3 billion.[45]

- The capacity to provide home care will be limited by declining family sizes, increasing rates of divorce and subsequently greater numbers of Australians living alone.[46] The number of people aged over 65 relative to the number of people of traditional working age will almost double, so that for 10 working age people there were 2 people over 65 in 2007 (20%), compared to 4 people over 65 for every 10 working age people (42%) in 2047. This will not only seriously compromise the ability to provide formal care for older Australians, but will undermine the capacity to raise taxes to fund these services. [47]

- It is projected that by 85 years of age, 62% of women and almost 50% of men will require residential aged care.[48] This leads to estimates that 337,500 aged care places will be needed by 2020, increasing to 464,000 places by 2030.[49] In 2015 there were 192,000 aged care places, meaning a 75% increase is required over 8 years.[50]

- An aged care bed costs on average $73,000 a year and is mostly subsidised by the Commonwealth.[51] Aged care funding is expected to double by 2055 as the per-person aged care expenditure increases from $620 to $2,000.[52]

- Increased longevity not only drives demand for supportive services and long term residential care, but also for shorter-term, emergency and inpatient medical care. The number of emergency department (ED) presentations across Australia increased by 6.5% from 2004-05 to 2013-14 for those 65 years and older.[53] This increase was even greater in the 85 years and older population, with an 8.3% increase in presentations.[54]

- A corollary of increasing ED presentations are increased hospital admissions, as elderly patients are more likely to be admitted and have a greater length of stay.[55] Public hospital expenditure is already on average four times greater in the 85 years and older group versus the average across all ages.[56] By 2050, the number of annual hospital bed days is expected to rise by 150% for those aged 60 and over and by 320% for Australians 85 years and over.[57]

As such, the health system — despite being at breaking point in providing care to thousands of older Australians — isn't providing the care they want and need, especially in the last years and months of people's lives. It is an unfortunate response that in light of the limitations of the health system, many Australians have come to fear 'natural' death and even fear ageing itself. It is even more unfortunate that palliative care, which can provide the holistic value-driven care Australians want at an efficient price, is not widely recognised or widely available — except for the exception to the rule, in the case of cancer patients.

Preferential treatment — more palliative care for cancer patients

For over a decade, there has been domestic and international evidence that cancer patients are overrepresented in receiving and accessing hospital and community palliative care services.[58] In Western Australia, 68% of people dying with cancer accessed specialised palliative care, compared to 8% of people dying from a non-cancer condition.[59] This is despite evidence that non-cancer patients are just as likely — if not more likely — to benefit from palliative care.

Due to advances in medicine and technology, many malignancies have transformed from being rapidly and devastatingly aggressive to chronic conditions. The 5-year survival in Australia from all cancers increased from 48% in 1984–1988 to 68% in 2009–2013.[60] Palliative care has worked hard to form an allegiance with oncology. There is a wealth of evidence to suggest that palliative care for cancer patients and their families improves outcomes including symptom control, anxiety and reduced hospitalisations.[61] Perhaps most influentially, a study comparing palliative care to standard care in patients with metastatic terminal lung cancer determined that those receiving palliative care not only had a better quality of life with less depression but survived longer, despite receiving less aggressive treatment.[62]

Cancer, unlike lung disease is far more likely to induce thoughts of mortality in patients and doctors — which has arguably led to the increased prescription of palliative care in these groups. There are a myriad of calculators, studies and guidelines pertaining to specific malignancies and the likelihood of five- and ten-year survival on the basis of numerous factors, such as patient age and the stage. Staging of malignancy is an established practice enabling doctors to recommend evidence informed therapy based on survival predictions.

As such, at diagnosis, prognosis is more likely to be discussed and this discussion is facilitated by a series of well-researched prognostic indicators. Early and more accurate prognostication presumably enables clinicians, patients and their families to have a more open discussion about the future and make informed decisions regarding palliation, life and death.

Even less palliative care for chronic disease sufferers

Despite being more prevalent, patients dying from non-malignant chronic conditions are less likely to have conversations with their doctors about their prognosis and survival, in part because their deaths are more unpredictable.[63] For example, using a mortality tool on a cohort of heart failure patients, the predicted median survival was two years while the actual median survival time was 21 days.[64]

Benefits have been shown for palliative care for patients suffering from a wide range of illnesses; including COPD, cystic fibrosis, pancreatitis, heart failure, osteoarthritis, end stage renal disease, HIV, and neurological conditions including stroke.[65] A study comparing various patients found that in the last three months of life, those suffering COPD were the least likely to be referred for palliative care (20%), after heart failure (34%), severe dementia (37%) and cancer (60%).[66] In a West Australian study of 1071 people who died in 2005-2006, 61% died in hospital and of these a greater proportion had a non-cancer diagnosis, and were from rural areas—demonstrating the characteristics pertaining to reduced access to palliative care.[67] The Victorian government estimates that at least 50% of people dying from diseases such as heart failure would benefit from palliative care.[68]

Heart failure has a complex and varied prognosis, in which patients are likely to experience a high burden of symptoms that progress with time e.g. breathlessness, anxiety and fatigue. It is a life-limiting illness and the population experiencing these symptoms is increasing—the lifetime risk of developing heart failure is around 20% for all adults and the mortality rate is higher than most cancers.[69] Studies suggest that many of these patients suffer poor quality of life exacerbated by frequent hospital admissions and would prefer their care to focus on 'comfort'.[70]

There are limited data demonstrating how many Australians with heart failure access palliative care. However, research suggests the experience of patients with heart failure is one of ignorance of their condition, poor communication with physicians, a focus predominately on curative treatment, poor end-of-life planning and symptom burden.[71] A study comparing patients with heart failure to those with cancer found those with non-malignant disease had more concerns around medications, social isolation and progressive loss, while receiving less palliative care and less co-ordinated care. This led researchers to conclude that "care for people with advanced progressive illnesses is currently prioritised by diagnosis rather than need."[72]

Throughout Australia the provision of palliative care for chronic disease sufferers is patchy at best. (This even includes end-stage kidney disease patients. [73 74 75 76]) Patients with cancer are more likely to receive and benefit from this care. Even among this population, palliative care is still arguably insufficient and untimely—however it is vastly superior to the care provided for non-cancer patients.

The palliative care gap in Australia fosters myths about death

Murtagh et al. (2011) determined that in high income countries up to 82% of people who die need palliative care. Last year, 159,000 people died in Australia. Applying Murtagh's statistic this equates to roughly 130,300 people requiring palliative care. In 2015-2016 only 14,300 patients received an MBS-subsidised palliative care medicine specialist service in Australia.[77]

Clearly there is a gaping chasm between the supply of, and the real demand for, palliative care in Australia. Lack of access to palliative care is a symptom of the larger structural problems in the Medicare system, which result in service gaps for chronic care, including palliative care. (See Box 6)

However, calls for more palliative care services are often based on the belief that too many Australians die in hospital. This applies a narrow definition of palliative care as purely 'end-of-life care', and distorts the broader benefits that good palliative care can provide for patients.

One measure of the inadequacy of palliative care in Australia is the purported statistic that most Australians would choose to die at home if they had a terminal illness, whereas most deaths in Australia actually occur in a hospital. According to one – much cited – survey, up to 70% of Australians would prefer to die at home, rather than in a hospital.[79] However, this statistic is unreliable, and its veracity has been questioned. Agar et al. (2008) in an Australian longitudinal study made sure to delineate between asking patients and their carers where they would prefer to be 'cared for' and where they would prefer to die. This is an important distinction—not made in most research of death preferences and demonstrated a trend toward many patients and their families ultimately preferring that death not to occur at home.[80] (See Box 7)

The notion that the problems associated with death and dying can be solved by allowing more Australians to die at home is an over-simplification. The myth that most people want to die at home—but don't—has also unhelpfully reinforced the popular fear that 'grim, distressing, painful and undignified' natural death in hospital should be avoided at all costs. These myths undermine the broader benefits that good palliative care can provide for patients.

Certainly, most Australians wish to age at home and the holistic approach of palliative care can facilitate this.[85] However, the majority of Australians are likely to continue to die in hospital, and in residential aged care facilities (RACFs). Death in hospital or a RACF is not the problem—death without palliative care is the real problem. Hospitals must be equipped to provide this type of care both in terms of workforce, culture and environment.

Similarly, palliative care should be readily available to thousands of elderly in RACFs. Demonising the idea of death occurring outside the home is a simplification of a bigger problem and unhelpfully adds to the growing premise that natural death in a hospital or RACF is undesirable.

Almost 50% of Australians die in hospital, and the reality is that most Australians are likely to continue to die in hospital. The focus of the debate about death and dying therefore needs to be broadened beyond the question of where patients die; because the real problem is not dying in hospital, but death without palliative care. The current provision of palliative care — as properly defined as care encompassing quality of life before death — in Australian hospitals and among residential aged care facilities is insufficient. The challenge is to ensure that hospitals offer greater access to palliative care to improve the quality of life before death for more Australians. Improved palliative care in these settings will not only contribute to better patient experiences and quality of life but will improve cost effectiveness both by preventing hospital admissions and also within hospitals by preventing unwanted interventions.

Box 6: : Medicare's Structural Flaws and the Palliative Care Gap

- It is well recognised within the Australian health policy debate that the chief systemic barrier to better outcomes and patient-centred care is the fragmentation of health services owing to the structural flaws in the complex funding and service arrangements that distinguish the Medicare system and the federal-state split in health responsibilities.[78]

- The federal government runs and funds the primary care part of Medicare. This oversees the Medical Benefits Scheme (MBS), the principal function of which is to pay benefits to meet or assist in covering the cost of fees mainly for GP care, medical imaging and diagnostic services, and other specialist ambulatory and inpatient attendances and procedures on a fee-for-service, on-demand, and open-ended basis. The federal government also gives state and territory governments a fixed amount of money each

---

year to partially fund the operation of public hospitals. Federal hospital funding is provided on condition that all Australians are entitled to receive 'free' public hospital care; but otherwise state and territory governments are responsible for hospital governance and administration.

- Jurisdictional complexity—with the result being that neither level of government is solely accountable for the entire healthcare needs of patients—distorts responsibilities and incentives in ways that partially account for the service gaps for chronic patients. Medicare provides access to separate sets of acute care services. It does not provide access to the full range of medical, pharmaceutical and allied healthcare that might ensure chronic conditions are properly managed to stop patients ending up in hospital. The fragmented and 'siloed' services patients receive is accentuated by the fact that aged care services are provided under yet another separate, federally-funded program.

- Palliative care is an important example of how there is no room within the current health (and aged care) system and its funding arrangement for flexible, innovative, integrated and comprehensive care. Instead these services are lost in the gap between what the federal government pays for and the state government funds. Such service gaps are also caused by the way current funding arrangements reward separate occasions of hospitalisation and GP activity over integrated community based multidisciplinary care – of which palliative care is an example.

- Hence the lack of access to palliative care services in Australia is a demonstration of how Medicare is not really a comprehensive health system but rather a doctor and hospital centric system. The biggest gaps exist when patients leave hospital or aren't in a GP clinic, i.e. where community based multidisciplinary palliative care should exist. However, in a fee-for-service system that rewards activity rather than outcomes, and is distinguished by siloed funding for hospital and non-hospital services, there is no incentive or funding available to provide truly patient-centred services. Palliative care is the square peg that doesn't fit into the round hole that is the Medicare system.

- Closing the palliative care 'gap' therefore requires addressing the inherent problems within Medicare, which rewards a rigid set of proscribed medical and hospital activity, rather than the delivery of holistic integrated care for dying Australians.

Box 7: The 70% myth

- The original statistic comes from a 2006 South Australian study that asked 2,652 individuals over the age of 15 "if they were dying of a terminal illness such as cancer or emphysema" where they would prefer to die.[81]

- Agar et al also found that preferences for place of care and place of death not only differed between patients and caregivers but changed for both—and not synchronously—over time. Their findings suggest a trend from home being the preferred place of care to an inpatient setting as death approaches. They concluded that asking patients 'where they want to die' is not sufficient in determining the nuances that exist as patients live before death, deteriorate and death becomes more acute.

- Previous studies have also concluded that relative to other considerations such as being pain free, place of death is a low priority for those who are dying.[82]

- Other studies have also considered caregiver perspectives and found that preference for home care reduced as death became more imminent (from 92% to 42%), for patients there was a similar decline (90% to 50%) in the last week of life.[83]

- There are numerous reasons for this change of mind; such as lack of carer or family resources, concerns about symptom control and comfort, the ability of family to provide care, concerns from patients about being a burden, as well as unexpected medical events or deteriorations.[84]

The lack of access to palliative care

The overwhelming majority of patients with a life-threatening illness do not receive specialist palliative care. There is unequitable access across the country and at present the likelihood of receiving palliative care is "nothing short of a lottery" and depends on your "location, diagnosis, cultural background, age, and (your) health professionals' education". [86] Many continue to miss out, and this includes not only patients but families so in need of bereavement support. It is ironic that the two places where most Australians die are arguably two places you are least likely to receive palliative care, acute hospitals and RACF.

Palliative care in Australian hospitals

Studies have identified that at least one fifth of hospitalised patients at any given time have needs that would benefit from palliative care.[87] Of hospital deaths, some data suggests up to 46% receive palliative care while other sources highlight as little as 3% receive palliative care.[88] However, the current hospital system does not readily enable this model of care to be delivered. Firstly, because treating clinicians do not consider, or are reluctant to refer to, palliative care—as seen in both metropolitan Melbourne and Sydney hospitals, where most patients in need were not referred for palliative care.[89] Secondly, even when palliative care is considered, there are barriers—sterile rooms, high turnover of busy staff, noisy atmosphere, restrictions on visitors, overcrowding and inadequate clinical training—to the provision of genuine, timely, considered care that incorporates a patient's family, their surroundings, their symptoms, and concerns.[90] It is not surprising that not all dying inpatients receive palliative care, and that even when they do it is often not best practice from a specialised palliative care team.[91]

Inpatient specialist palliative care not only ensures a more comfortable period of living for patients and their families before death, but is also more cost effective. An Australian study corroborated by international findings suggests that palliative care associated cost reduction in mean total cost for an episode of terminal care was $6,662 for cancer patients and $7,477 for other patients. There were also savings in private hospitals, although they provided less palliative care.[92] These savings largely came about due to a reduction in ICU admissions and operative procedures. In the US, similar cost savings have been found and it is estimated that $84 million to $252 million could be saved annually in New York State alone if all hospitals with more than 150 beds had a specialist palliative care service—and their services were utilised.[93]

Palliative care in residential aged care facilities

Access to palliative care for residents in aged care facilities has been shown to increase the likelihood of dying at home rather than hospital.[94] However, older Australians without cancer from aged care facilities are the least likely to receive palliative care.[95] In Australia (2015-16), only 9,144 aged care residents had an Aged Care Funding Instrument (ACFI) assessment that indicated the need for palliative care—this corresponds to roughly 4% of residents being assessed as requiring palliative care. This must be a gross underestimate and demonstrates a failure to recognise the needs of residents, especially given that over a third of residents die within a year of admission.[96] Previous studies have determined that palliative care in Australian RACFs is sub optimal—contributing to poor pain management, unwarranted hospital admissions, and resident and family upset.[97]

Experts speculate the ACFI is misrepresentative because the addition of palliative care needs for some residents does not add to their overall remuneration. Additionally, the requirements for a RACF to claim for palliative care may be unachievable, as care must be provided by a capable Registered Nurse (RN) usually under direction from a GP or palliative care specialist.[98] Moreover, RACFs are encouraged to claim for palliative care when a patient is terminal; however, the benefits patients and families glean from palliative care can be seen much earlier in a patient's life than the last few hours or days.

Up to 95% of residents experience an emergency transfer each year.[99] On presenting to ED, these patients are usually unwell with multiple complex comorbidities, and are at a high risk of firstly being admitted but then suffering in-hospital complications including pressure ulcers and delirium.[100] Up to 80% experience invasive interventions and 34% die in hospital.[101]

There is evidence that some emergency department presentations and hospital admissions are the direct result of a lack of community palliative care resources.[102] Having expressed a wish to die at home, having a palliative 'treatment goal' and receiving palliative care by a GP, reduces the likelihood of being hospitalised in the last three months of life.[103] Patients who are either unable to access palliative care services at home or unable to access services acutely i.e. after hours, are more likely to be transferred by ambulance to hospital.[104]

Hospitalisations account for the significantly higher health care costs per person in the last six months of life. In a recent study of decedents from NSW with and without cancer in their last six months of life, decedents with cancer visited the ED once, had three hospital admissions, participated in 90 clinician visits/procedures and were prescribed 41 medications at an average cost of $30 001 per decedent, roughly $4000 more on average than patients without cancer.[105] Worryingly only 10% of the cohort (total = 4271) dying from cancer and 1% of the comparison non cancer cohort (total = 3072) received a palliative care service whilst they were in hospital. Persons who died outside of a hospital had at least 42% lower overall costs compared to those who died in hospital.

A palliative care program, including an interdisciplinary approach to home based end-of-life care, provided to over 558 patients in the US, demonstrated fewer emergency department visits, days in hospital, and clinician visits than those in the control group. There was a 45% decrease in costs in the group receiving palliative care.[106] Community based in-home palliative care is more likely to be associated with significantly increased patient satisfaction and a reduction in the utilisation of medical services, lending itself to be both a valuable patient centred approach as well as a cost effective one.[107] However, access to in-house palliative care is also dependent largely on location, with lower socioeconomic areas being under serviced.[108] Of the palliative care related public hospital separations more people are from lower socioeconomic areas (26 per 100,000 population) than those living in higher socioeconomic areas (14 per 100,000 population) — suggesting higher socioeconomic patients are more likely to be receiving in home palliative care services and die at home.[109]

Another challenge: the funding of palliative care in Australia

There is significant variability in the provision of palliative care across facilities and across the country. Patients with cancer are more likely to receive palliative care, but even this cohort is under-serviced. Access to palliative care is even more limited for marginalised groups such as

Indigenous Australians, patients with a disability and those living rurally. As determined by the Grattan Institute report in 2014,[110] palliative care services in Australia are fragmented and inadequate in supply. This was corroborated this year by the Auditor General of NSW stating that "NSW Health has a limited understanding of the quantity and quality of palliative care services across the state, which reduces its ability to plan for future demand and the workforce needed to deliver it."[111]

Even within a large tertiary hospital in Melbourne, less than half the patients requiring palliative care were referred for such services—despite the fact that when received, palliative care was associated with improved end-of-life medication orders, improved communication with patients and families, and increased cessation of futile treatment and interventions.[112]

In a 2010-2013, a parliamentary inquiry committee determined that there is much inconsistency in the standard of palliative care delivered in Australia and this is likely due to the complexity of the funding framework (See Box 8).[113]The funding of palliative care services is varied within states and across the country.

However, differences in service provision are difficult to describe, given the lack of data regarding access and outcomes of palliative care nationwide. The paucity of data to assess the provision of palliative care services extends to admitted patients and patients in the community and primary care settings. This contributes to a failure of accountability within the sector, an inability to plan for the future and has resulted in the ad hoc nature of service provision.[114] Over a decade ago, a study in England determined if patients who had non-malignant disease were provided with palliative care at the rate cancer patients were, it would mean a 79% increase in the caseload for palliative care services.[115] Meeting unmet needs for palliative care in Australia—including providing for marginal groups such as Aboriginal and Torres Strait Islanders—would certainly raise significant workforce issues (See Box 9).

Box 8: The variety of funding Hospital funding

- The majority of palliative care is provided by the public hospital sector and can be funded under the Australian National Sub-Acute and Non-Acute Patient Classification (AN-SNAP).[116]

- AN-SNAP was established as part of activity based funding in 2013 after the National Health Reform Agreement in 2011. The IHPA has recently released AN-SNAP Version 4 to better reflect current and evolving clinical practice in subacute services, and has introduced paediatric classes for palliative care.

- Some public hospitals use sub-acute funding to subsidise palliative care provided by staff specialists within the hospital. However, sub-acute funding is packaged, and it is up to the discretion of the state/hospital to determine how much is spent on palliative care. For example, in 2009-2010 "Of its $39,973 sub-acute funding South Australia committed $11,970 to palliative care. On the other hand, Queensland allocated none of the sub-acute funding to palliative care."[117]

- There have been calls to separate palliative care from the sub-acute funding, however this was recently rejected by the Australian government.

- Other inpatient services receive block funding to provide inpatient palliative care under the Health Services Act 1997 and service level agreements. Often these organisations also provide community care and in-reach services (e.g. to RACFs). Specialist funding • Specialist palliative care physicians can claim under the Medicare Benefits Scheme. In 2015-2016 $5.6 million was paid in benefits for palliative care specialist services for 74,300 occasions. This has increased by 60% over the past five years, reflecting the significant trend towards the increasing need for palliative care.[118]

- Importantly, palliative care can be provided—and should be provided—by other specialist clinicians such as geriatricians and oncologists. However, they are unable to claim care as a palliative care related service under the MBS.

- There are no palliative care Medicare Benefit Schedule (MBS) specific items that can be used by GPs. Instead GPs use other items to deliver palliative care, such as a GP management plan. This remuneration likely underestimates the complexity of these patients and the time taken for appropriate care to be given to them and their families.

- It is consequently impossible to quantify the amount of palliative care being performed by general practitioners, or the associated costs. Not only does this make it difficult for policy makers to assess and predict the needs for the future, inadequate remuneration is a disincentive to providing this care.

- Providing palliative care is an essential skill for GPs and the need for this will only increase. GPs should be encouraged to upskill and deliver this essential care by at the very least having an identifiable and separate MBS items to claim for this care. RACF funding • RACFs claim for palliative care under the ACFI, which likely underrepresents the real need for palliative care.

- The paucity of palliative care services in RACFs under the current funding model may well be due to the inadequacy of GPs and a lack of access to specialists including nurses. Registered nurses (RNs) are essential to the delivery of palliative care within RACFs.

- Many RACFs cannot provide palliative care because of GP skill and a lack of RNs. In 2016, RNs made up 15% of the residential aged care workforce—down from 21% in 2003 despite an increase in the number of residents. One does not have to look far to appreciate how understaffed RACFs are. • All RACFs should be capable of providing palliative care. Informal care • Informal carers do not receive training or supervision and are estimated to provide at least $6.5 billion worth of care in Australia per year.[119]

- Carers are often spouses—who may be older than the patients themselves—or other family, friends and neighbours. Most are co-resident, spending 24 hours a day with the patient. Even if people do not die at home, 90% of palliative care patients spend the majority of their time living before death at home supported by a carer.[120] The needs of carers cannot be overestimated—physically, economically, socially and psychologically—in light of the fact that the person they are investing so much time, energy and emotion in will ultimately pass away. • The cost of paying for 24 hours' worth of active care in NSW is roughly $1,332.00 per 24hrs, not including weekend or public holiday rates, adding up to $9,324 per week.[121]

- There are increasing numbers of older adults living alone, and—together with reduced family sizes and increasing work place commitments—there is little likelihood that the amount of this informal care will continue to meet the needs of our ageing population.

> **Box 9: The palliative care workforce; underfunded and understaffed**
>
> - In 2015, specialist palliative care physicians made up around 1 in 140 (0.7%) of the employed medical specialists in Australia.[122] This corresponds to around 213 palliative care specialists working in Australia, compared to 1,040 cardiologists and 511 geriatricians. There were 85 doctors in palliative care training in 2015 compared to 177 cardiology trainees.[123]
>
> - In 2015, the majority of palliative care physicians were female and worked in major city hospitals. Across Australia there were 0.9 FTE specialist palliative physicians per 100,000 population and this ranged from none in the ACT to 1.8 in Tasmania.[124] There has been a roughly 50% increase in the number of specialist palliative care physicians since 2012. Nationally, there were 12.0 FTE palliative care nurses per 100,000 population in 2015 making up 1.1% of employed nurses.[125]
>
> - In 2003 Palliative Care Australia (PCA) recommended 1.5 FTE palliative care physicians per 100,000 population for the reasonable provision of palliative care services nationwide. 14 years later, the gap is ongoing.
>
> - One solution is a greater emphasis being placed on palliative care throughout the academic life of a doctor. Unfortunately, there is still inadequacy in palliative care training reported by physicians, surgeons, medical students and advanced trainees.[126]
>
> - But it is not only doctors who provide palliative care. To face the challenges of a declining workforce combined with an ageing population, health professionals are going to need to step beyond the traditional boundaries of their disciplines.
>
> - A recent proposition for nurse practitioners to prescribe palliative care medications was 'supported in principle' but is ultimately under the jurisdiction of the Australian Health Practitioner Regulation Agency (AHPRA) and likely to be a difficult reform.

Palliative Policy—perfect on paper but inadequate in practice

Palliative care policy in Australia is supposedly guided by The *National Palliative Care Strategy 2010: Supporting Australians to Live Well at the End of Life. This replaced the first* National Palliative Care Strategy: *A National Framework for Palliative Care Service Development 2000* which began in 1998. The more recent strategy is actioned by the National Palliative Care

Projects (NPCP). These projects are unique, ranging across Australia from small local projects to multi-institutional collaborations. Each received an array of government funding as they were seen to align with the goals identified in the 2010 Strategy.

A recent review of the strategy and the associated NPCPs revealed some successes and significant limitations.[127] Pointedly, the strategy itself was often not actually identified among local- and state-based professionals or plans — leading to duplication, misalignment and diffusion of responsibility. For example, in NSW the Agency for Clinical Innovation Palliative Care Network was established in 2012 to "drive continuous improvement in palliative and end-of-life care for all people approaching or reaching the end of their life in NSW" as instructed by the *NSW Government plan to increase access to palliative care 2012-2016* with $35 million worth of funding.

This strategy is yet to be successfully implemented, reviewed and critiqued. The Clinical Excellence Commission also in NSW has an end of life program, and similarly most other states and territories have their own palliative care plan. Whether or not any of these plans or programs have been comprehensively realised remains to be seen, and likely contributes to the variation in services.

Advanced care plans demonstrate that conversations about end-of-life care result in better outcomes and improve clinician decision-making. Advanced care directives (ACD) are tangible documents that form part of advanced care planning — which involves conversations with families and clinicians. The laws underpinning ACDs differ across Australia.[128] A national survey found that 14% of the population has an ACD,[129] while other studies have revealed in NSW only 5% of residential aged care residents had an ACD.[130]

The use, understanding and legal framework of ACDs across the country are extraordinarily varied. The legal ramifications are poorly understood, and the directives themselves are often misplaced, clouded with uncertainty and poorly documented[131]. The government needs to take responsibility for creating a clear and comprehensive policy and legal framework on a national level regarding advanced care planning.

A recent review of palliative care within NSW led to the recommendation that NSW Health needs an "integrated palliative and end-of-life care policy framework". More importantly it needs to implement this framework.[132]

How to improve life before death?
Policy makers, doctors and society

Policy makers must move on from paying lip service to palliative care and start by bolstering the workforce. Funding needs to be directed towards increasing the number of RNs and doctors in particular to provide this care nationwide. Seemingly a simple solution, the likelihood is this will have significant implications for the cost of the system as a whole going forward, given the cost effectiveness of a palliative care framework. Australian governments need to provide leadership to address the dual ethical and economic challenges of promoting access to cost-effective and quality of life-enhancing palliative care services. State and federal governments should also consider adopting an 'investment approach' to palliative care provision that would ensure Australia finally sees implementation of the recommendations of the innumerable reports and reviews calling for expanded availability.

Undertaking a longitudinal actuarial study of the lifetime costs of chronic disease in the latter and last stages of life without palliative care will help inform decisions about service and funding redesigns that will lead to greater provision and access to cost-effective palliative services. Understanding the real costs of the existing unintegrated, reactionary 'end of life' care across the fragmented health and aged care systems would help encourage rational policy responses from federal and state governments to re-orientate the health system away from simply reactive, life-protracting care towards holistic, person-centred care. This could drive a national approach to palliative care, encompassing even a joint federal-state funding instrument. State and federal governments should also think boldly about ways to ensure comprehensive access, integrated services, accountability and choice. This should involve exploring consumer-centred and commissioning-based models of palliative care that focus on "improving outcomes and delivering quality services, regardless of organisational boundaries and constraints"[133] with the interests of the patient and their families at the centre.

The medical profession must do better

While the policy challenges are real and significant, the delivery of timely and quality palliative care will ultimately depend on the willingness and ability of the doctors to identify and refer patients. Expanding access to palliative services will therefore require leadership from the Australian medical profession. This must entail altering the current scope of clinical practices that erect barriers to access by making doctors disinclined to discuss patient's end-of-life preferences, and identify and refer patients, or practise palliative care themselves. It is an unfortunate reality that despite decades of research, policies, funding and public campaigns, the rest of the medical profession has been alarmingly reticent to discuss patient values and goals, and either provide palliative care or refer them for specialist palliative care in a timely manner. A study by the Royal Australian College of Physicians revealed "only 17 per cent of physicians believed doctors were always aware of their patients' death-related preferences."[134]

The majority of general practitioners completing a survey, mostly from metropolitan Melbourne (n=56), did not routinely discuss end-of-life care or advanced care planning with their patients.[135] A 2016 study of 178 patients with advanced cancer discovered that only 9 (5%) had a completely accurate understanding of their illness.[136] Other studies have suggested that patients receive more information about their illness from other patients in the waiting room than from their doctor.

Doctors need to start ensuring care — for elderly patients, at the very least — is made in partnership with patients and their families with their overall goals in mind. All doctors should be capable of providing palliative care — even at the same time as curative care — and more need to be willing to refer patients for specialist services and do so before the terminal phase of life. Even studies demonstrating how few doctors discuss end of life preferences highlight the narrow-minded focus on death, instead of life before death.

Palliative care must become integrated into subspecialty training. And, just as resuscitation skills are taught and mandated, the same should apply to having 'difficult' conversations with patients and their families. More needs to be done to alleviate the lack of confidence within the medical community to discuss an issue that should be core business. Having discussions about life and death will become imperative and doctors need to start fulfilling their individual and societal obligation to have these conversations and — more importantly—provide this care. This expertise must extend beyond the realm of oncology and metropolitan Sydney.

Palliative care is much more than ensuring a 'good death' and should be provided based on a patient's symptomatology and their goals for life. The medical profession's engagement with the task of repositioning palliative care in the health system and placing the focus on life before death should be driven by an awareness of the pressing ethical challenges associated with death and dying. The alternative prospect, by default, of radical changes to clinical ethics and practice will place an already under-serviced and undervalued 'old and dying' population at greater vulnerability. Closing the 'palliative care gap' between supply and demand will also require greater community awareness of the benefits of palliative care. Informing more Australians about what palliative care is and what it can do—and how it can fix the deficiencies in the health system that foster the fear of a 'horrible death'—is also crucial to drive overdue policy change.

The Australian public deserve better

Australians perceive that the experience of ageing, health and death is changing. However, despite the best attempts of a series of programs and lobby groups to encourage Australians to discuss ageing, death and dying, this domain has been overwhelmed by those pushing an agenda of fear and personal stories. In light of the limitations within the health system explored here, and the lack of palliative care, this message is dominating the minds of those approaching old age. Palliative care is a welcome solution to the visible deficiencies in the system but is unable to receive the attention it deserves.

Doctors already wary of the increasingly informed patient must put their pride and pedestals away and be willing to engage with patients as partners. Together, there is much common ground to be found—and the more common this practice becomes the easier it will be to make better decisions about patient care. As an American doctor forecasting the future of medicine put it:

> The more patients and families become empowered, shaping their care, the better that care becomes, and the lower the costs. Clinicians, and those who train them, should learn how to ask less, "What is the matter with you?" and more, "What matters to you?"[138]

Communities—and by extension, society—need to provide options for older people who seek supportive care to remain as active as possible. Whether that be by volunteering, engaging in work, being able to travel or contribute in some way. The common thought that one would 'rather die than be in a nursing home' (or pursue more radical alternatives to forestall natural death) should challenge policy makers and doctors to ensure more attractive options are available for an increasing number of older Australians to die well and live better.

Conclusion

Australians have for many years now experienced great improvements in health. We are living longer than ever before, and most of our lives are spent in good health. Conditions that used to kill more quickly, and at younger ages, have been replaced by chronic disease—and lower death rates show how we reach greater ages despite a greater burden of disease.

This progression in health and change in illness can be largely attributed to public health, subspecialisation and the advancements in modern medicine. However, this has meant a changed experience of death for many Australians and their families. After living well with chronic diseases for many years, they find themselves facing a downward trajectory in health. At this time, many are let down by the health system set in its 'treat and cure' ways. The experience for many Australians and their families is one of confusion, multiple visits to doctors, clinics, hospitals, ambulances with little in the way of holistic care. This eventually results more often than not in an acute hospital visit that leads to death without palliative care—and occasionally, without an awareness that one was even dying.

The health system's failure to adapt to the changing nature of ageing and death, and provide quality care to the elderly and dying, has meant this time of life has become shrouded in myths of desolation and indignity. The inability of the health system to provide palliative care generally has raised an unhelpful focus on where people die, rather than how they die and how they lived prior to death. These assumptions, together with a societal bent for youth and independence, has created a climate where old age and death is dreaded.

Palliative care is holistic value- driven care that is patient- and family-centred, pre-emptory and perfectly situated to support chronic disease sufferers in their later years of life. Palliative care is also cost-effective care that reduces hospital admissions, means patients live at home (including RACFs) longer, and in hospital prevents dissatisfaction and over-treatment. This amalgamates to palliative care being an efficient use of resources, especially in light of the pattern of disease among our ageing population. More so, it is better care—and care that older Australians want and deserve.

However, in Australia access to palliative care is limited. Preferentially, services are provided for patients dying of cancer. However, diagnosis should not dictate access to palliative care—as patients suffering from all types of chronic disease benefit from palliative care. Patients who live rurally, have a disability or are Indigenous, have even less access to palliative care. However, alarmingly, so do those who die in hospital and in RACFs. Patients are likely to continue to die in hospital and RACFs from many other diseases apart from cancer, and these patients also warrant access to palliative care. At present, it's the lucky Australians who receive palliative care.

A palliative care policy is required that ensures comprehensive access, integrated services, accountability and choice: this is a public health issue, as well as an ethical and economic issue. A consumer-centred or commissioning approach, as recommended by the Productivity Commission, could be used to drive reform, improve access, and increase quality across the social services sector. Embracing an investment approach would also highlight the cost benefits of widespread palliative care in light of an ever increasing older population.

Expanding access to palliative care in Australia will ensure that older Australians look forward to quality of life before death, and the choice of palliative care at the end of life, no matter where they die.

Endnotes

1 Sammut, J., Thomas, G., Seaton, P. (2016). MEDI-VATION: 'Health Innovation= Communities' for Medicare Payment and Service Reform.

2 Productivity Commission, 2017. Inquiry report no. 84. Shifting the dial, Canberra.

3 Productivity Commission, 2016. Introducing Competition and Informed User Choice into Human Services: Identifying Sectors for Reform, Preliminary Findings Report, Canberra.

4 https://governmentnews.com.au/2017/08/palliative-care-nsw-health-must-improve/

5 Harper, I., Anderson, P., McCluskey, S., O'Bryan. (2015). Competition Policy Review. Commonwealth of Australia.

6 Parikh R.B, Kirch R.A, Smith T.J, Temel J.S. (2013).Early specialty palliative care—translating data in oncology into practice. *NEJM*369: 2347-51;Christakis N.A, & Iwashyna T.J. (2003). The health impact of health care on families: a matched cohort study of hospice use by decedents and mortality outcomes in surviving, widowed spouses. *Social Science and Medicine*57: 465-475.; Temel, et al. (2010). Early Palliative Care for Patients with Metastatic Non–Small-Cell Lung Cancer, *NEJM*; 363:733-742

7 WHO. Definition of Palliative Care: http://www.who.int/cancer/palliative/definition/en/

8 Morrison, R.S. (2013). Models of palliative care delivery in the United States. *Current opinion in supportive and palliative care.* 7(2):201-206.

9 Centre to Advance Palliative Care. (2015). America's Care of Serious Illness 2015 State-By-State Report Card on Access to Palliative Care in Our Nation's Hospitals.

10 Centre to Advance Palliative Care. (2015). America's Care of Serious Illness 2015 State-By-State Report Card on Access to Palliative Care in Our Nation's Hospitals.

11 al-Awamer, A. (2015). Physician-assisted suicide is not a failure of palliative care. *Canadian Family Physician*.61(12):1039-1040; St Vincent's Health Australia. (2017). Palliative and end of life care; Position Statement.

12 al-Awamer, A. (2015). Physician-assisted suicide is not a failure of palliative care. *Canadian Family Physician*.61(12):1039-1040

13 Monforte-Royo C, Villavicencio-Chávez C, Tomás-Sábado J, Mahtani-Chugani V, Balaguer A. (2012). What Lies behind the Wish to Hasten Death? A Systematic Review and Meta-Ethnography from the Perspective of Patients. PLoS ONE7(5): e37117

14 Dierckx de Casterle, B., Verpoort, C., De Bal, N., & Gastmans, C. (2006). Nurses' views on their involvement in euthanasia: a qualitative study in Flanders (Belgium). *Journal of Medical Ethics*; 32:187-192.

15 Unpublished data from Hudson, P., Hudson, R., Philip, J., Boughey, M., Kelly, B., & Hertogh, C. (2015). Legalizing physician-assisted suicide and/or euthanasia: Pragmatic implications. *Palliative and Supportive Care*, 13(05), 1399-1409.

16 ANZSPM (Australian and New Zealand Society of Palliative Medicine) 2008. Defining the meaning of the terms consultant physician in palliative medicine and palliative medicine specialist. Canberra: ANZSPM

17 AIHW. (2017). Life Expectancy and death.

18 Intergenerational Report, 2015

19 Intergenerational Report, 2015

20 Intergenerational Report, 2015

21 Intergenerational Report, 2015

22 Productivity Commission. (2013). An Ageing Australia: Preparing for the Future.

23 ABS. (1998). Population Projections, Australia, 1997 to 2051

24 ABS. (2013). Population Projections, Australia, 2012 (base) to 2101.

25 Shryock & Siegal. et al. (1976).The methods and materials of demography. New York; Academic Press.

26 ABS. (1998). Population Projections, Australia, 1997 to 2051

27 ABS. (2017). Deaths, Australia, 2016.

28 ABS. (2017). Deaths, Australia, 2016.

29 ABS. (2013). Population Projections, Australia, 2012 (base) to 2101

30 ABS. (2016). Causes of Death, Australia, 2015

31 http://www.smh.com.au/national/health/this-chart-shows-how-you-will-probably-die-and-its-changed-a-lot-in-100-years-20160509-gopmgh.html

32 Cassel, C., & Reuben, D. (2011). Specialization, Subspecialization, and Subsubspecialization in Internal Medicine. NEJM 364:1169-1173

33 AIHW. Australia's Health 2016.

34 AIHW. (2006). Mortality over the twentieth century in Australia Trends and patterns in major causes of death

35 AIHW. (2017). Trends in Death.

36 University of Sydney. BEACH. (2015). Care of Older People in Australian General Practice

37 Dept. Health & Ageing & Medicines Australia joint report. (2013). Trends in and drivers of Pharmaceutical Benefits Scheme expenditure

38 National Commission of Audit. Towards Responsible Government The Report of the National Commission of Audit – Phase One.; Linjakumpu T, et al. (2002). Use

of medications and polypharmacy are increasing among the elderly. *Journal Clinical Epidemiology*, 55(8):809–817.

39 Wise J. (2013). Polypharmacy: a necessary evil. *BMJ*.;347

40 AIHW. Australia's Health 2016.

41 Productivity Commission Research Paper. (2008). Trends in Aged Care Services: some implications

42 Langton, J.M., et al. (2016). Health service use and costs in the last 6 months of life in elderly decedents with a history of cancer: a comprehensive analysis from a health payer perspective. *British Journal of Cancer*, 114, 1293-1302.

43 In 2013–2014 and 2015–2016, almost 50% of Australians died in hospital. Even within the 108 specialist palliative care services, who submitted data to the Palliative Care Outcomes Collaboration (PCOC) in the year 2016, 72% of patients died in hospital.43 The remaining 50% of Australians likely die in RACFs, or at home, however there is a lack of data clearly demonstrating where Australians die. Palliative Care Outcomes Collaboration. (2017). National results for July – December 2016 Detailed report.

44 AIHW. (2013). The desire to age in place among older Australians.

45 Access Economics (2015). The economic value of informal care in Australia in 2015.

46 ABS. (2015). Household and Family Projections, Australia, 2011 to 2036

47 Productivity Commission Research Paper. (2008). Trends in Aged Care Services: some implications

48 Cullen, D. (2007). The financial impact of entering aged care. Australasian Journal of Ageing 26(3): 145–7.; Ergas, H. (2009). Providing *Aged Care: The Case for Reform.*

49 Ergas, H. (2009). Providing Aged Care: The Case for Reform.

National Health and Hospitals Reform Commission (NHHRC) 2009, 'Interim report—A healthier future for all Australians'.

50 Ergas, H. (2009). Providing Aged Care: The Case for Reform.

51 Ergas, H. (2009). Providing Aged Care: The Case for Reform; https://www.agedcare101.com.au/aged-care/working-out-your-finances/understand-financial-basics

52 Intergenerational Report, 2015

53 Australian Institute of Health and Welfare 2016. Australia's health 2016. Australia's health series no. 15. Cat. no. AUS 199. Canberra: AIHW

54 Australian Institute of Health and Welfare 2016. Australia's health 2016. Australia's health series no. 15. Cat. no. AUS 199. Canberra: AIHW

55 Katelaris, A. (2011). Time to rethink end-of-life care. Medical Journal *of Australia, 194(11), 563.*

56 Intergenerational Report, 2015

57 Schofield, D.J., & Earnest, A. (2006). Demographic change and the future demand for public hospital care in Australia, 2005 to 2050. Australian Health Review, 30(4), 507-515.

58 Rosenwax, L.K., & McNamara, B.A. (2006). Who receives specialist palliative care in Western Australia- and who misses out. *Palliative Medicine, 20*, p 439-445.

Bhatnagar S, Prabhakar H. (2012) Palliative care beyond oncology!. *Indian J Palliative Care*,18:85-6.

59 Rosenwax, L.K., & McNamara, B.A. (2006). Who receives specialist palliative care in Western Australia- and who misses out. *Palliative Medicine, 20*, p 439-445

60 AIHW. (2017). Cancer in Australia 2017.

61 Higginson, I. J., & Evans, C. J. (2010). What is the evidence that palliative care teams improve outcomes for cancer patients and their families?. *The Cancer Journal, 16*(5), 423-435.

62 Temel, J.S, et al. (2010). Early palliative care for patients with metastatic non-small-cell lung cancer. NEJM.19;363(8):733-42

63 Beernaert, K., et al.,. (2013). Referral to palliative care in COPD and other chronic diseases: A population-based study. *Respiratory Medicine*, 107 (11), 1731-1739.

64 Bakitas, M., et al. (2013). Palliative Care Consultations for Heart Failure Patients: How Many, When, and Why? *Journal Cardiac Failure* 19(3): 193–201.

65 Bhatnagar S, & Prabhakar H. (2012) Palliative care beyond oncology!. *Indian J Palliatiave Care*,18:85-6.

66 Beernaert, K., et al.,. (2013). Referral to palliative care in COPD and other chronic diseases: A population-based study. *Respiratory Medicine*, 107 (11), 1731-1739.

67 Rosenwax, L., McNamara, B., Murray, K., McCabe, R., Aoun, S., & Currow, D. (2011). Hospital and emergency department use in the last year of life: a baseline for future modifications to end-of-life care. *Medical Journal of Australia,194*, p570–573

68 Victorian department of Health: Strengthening palliative care: policy and strategic directions 2011-2015.

69 Bakitas, M., et al.,. (2013). Palliative Care Consultations for Heart Failure Patients: How Many, When, and Why? ;*Journal Cardiac Failure* 19(3): 193–201.Bui, A.L., Horwich, T.B., & Fonarow, G.C. (2011). Epidemiology and risk profile of heart failure. *Nature Reviews Cardiology*, 8;30-41.

70 Levenson JW, McCarthy EP, Lynn J, Davis RB, Phillips RS. (2000). The last six months of life for patients with congestive heart failure. J Am Geriatr Soc. 2000 May; 48(5 Suppl):S101-9., Juenger J, Schellberg D, Kraemer S, et al. (2002). Health related quality of life in patientafs with congestive heart failure: comparison with other chronic diseases and relation to functional variables. Heart, 87:235–241., Cowie MR, Fox KF, Wood DA, Metcalfe C, Thompson SG, Coats AJ, et al. (2002). Hospitalization of patients with heart failure: a population-based study. Eur Heart J, 23:842–845.

71 Wotton, K., Borbasi, S., & Redden, M. (2005). When all else has failed: Nurses; perception of factors influencing palliative care for patients with end-stage heart failure. *Journal cardiovascular Nursing* 20(1); 18-25.; Lindtworth, K., et al. (2015). Living with and dying from advanced heart failure: understanding the needs of older patients at the end of life. *BMC Geriatrics*, 15:125.

72 Murray, S.A., et al. (2002). Dying of lung cancer or cardiac failure: prospective qualitative interview study of patients and their carers in the community. *BMJ*, 325;929.

73 Murtagh, F.E., et al.. (2011). Trajectories of illness in stage 5 chronic kidney disease: a longitudinal study of patients symptoms and concerns in the last year of life. *Clinical Journal of the American Society of Nephrology*, 6 (7)l 1580-90.

74 Fassett, R.G. et al. (2011). Palliative care in end-stage kidney disease. *Nephrology*, 16;4-12.; Murtagh, F.E., et al.. (2011). Trajectories of illness in stage 5 chronic kidney disease: a longitudinal study of patients symptoms and concerns in the last year of life. *Clinical Journal of the American Society of Nephrology*, 6 (7)l 1580-90.

75 Fassett, R.G. et al. (2011). Palliative care in end-stage kidney disease. *Nephrology*, 16;4-12

76 Fassett, R.G. et al. (2011). Palliative care in end-stage kidney disease. *Nephrology*, 16;4-12.

77 AIHW. (2017). Palliative care services in Australia

78 Jeremy Sammut, Medi-Value: health insurance and service innovation in Australia -implications for the future of Medicare, Research Report 14, (Sydney: The Centre for Independent Studies, 2016).

79 Foreman et al. (2006). Factors predictive of preferred place of death in the general population of South Australia. *European Associate for Palliative Care*, 20(4), p447-453.

80 Agar, M., et al. (2008). Preference for place of care and place of death in palliative care: are these different questions? *Palliative Medicine*, 22.; Hoare, S., Morris, Z.S, Kelly, M.P., Kuhn, I., & Barclay, S. (2015). Do patients want to die at home? A systematic review of the UK literature, focused on missing preferences for place of death. PLoS ONE 10(11).

81 Foreman et al. (2006). Factors predictive of preferred place of death in the general population of South Australia. European Associate *for Palliative Care, 20(4), p447-453.*

82 Steinhauser, K.E. et al. (2000). Factors considered important at the end of life by patients, family, physicians, and other care providers. JAMA, 284(19):2476-2482.

83 Hinton, J. (1994). Can home care maintain an acceptable quality of life for patients with terminal cancer and their relatives? Palliative Medicine, *8(3); 183-96.*

84 Ireland, A. (2017). Access to palliative care services during a terminal hospital episode reduces intervention rates and hospital costs: a database study of 19 707 elderly patients dying in hospital, 2011–2015. Internal Medicine *Journal*, accepted 2017.

85 AIHW. (2013). The desire to age in place among older Australians

86 Hudson, P., Hudson, R., Philip, J., Boughey, M., Kelly, B., & Hertogh, C. (2015). Legalizing physician-assisted suicide and/or euthanasia: Pragmatic implications. *Palliative and Supportive Care*, 13(05), 1399-1409.

87 Gott, M., Frey,R., Raphael, D., O'Callaghan, A., Robinson, J., & Boyd, M. (2013). Palliative care need and management in the acute hospital setting: a census of one New Zealand Hospital. *BMC Palliative Care*, 12;15

88 AIHW. (2017). Palliative care services in Australia; Langton, J.M., et al. (2016). Health service use and costs in the last 6 months of life in elderly decedents with a history of cancer: a comprehensive analysis from a health payer perspective. *British Journal of Cancer*, 114, 1293-1302.

89 Huong Canh Le, B &Watt, J. (2010). Care of the dying in Australia's busiest hospital: benefits of palliative care consultation and methods to enhance access. *Journal of Palliative Medicine*. 13(7): 855-860; Unpublished data from Sydney Metropolitan hospital.

90 Virdun, C., Luckett, T., Davidson, P.M., & Philips, J. (2015). Dying in the hospital setting: A systematic review of quantitative studies identifying the elements of end-of-life care that patients and their families rank as being most important. *Palliative Medicine*, 29(9):774-96.

91 Gott, M., Ahmedzai, S., & Wood, C. (2001). How many inpatients at an acute hospital have palliative care needs? Comparing the perspectives of medical and nursing staff. *Palliative Medicine*, 15(6), 451-460.; Huong Canh Le, B. H. & Watt, J. N. (2010). Care of the dying in Australia's busiest hospital: benefits of palliative care consultation and methods to enhance access. *Journal of Palliative Medicine*. 13(7): 855-860

92 Ireland, A. (2017). Access to palliative care services during a terminal hospital episode reduces intervention rates and hospital costs: a database study of 19 707 elderly patients dying in hospital, 2011–2015. *Internal Medicine Journal*, accepted 2017.

93 Morrison, et al. (2011). Palliative care consultation teams cut hospitals costs for Medicaid beneficiaries. *Health Affairs*, 30(3). 454-463

94 Houttekier, D., Cohen, J., Van den Block, L., Bossuyt, N & Deliens, L. (2010). Involvement of Palliative Care Services Strongly Predicts Place of Death in Belgium. *Journal of Palliative Medicine*, 13(12): 1461-1468.

95 Rosenwax, L.K., & McNamara, B.A. (2006). Who receives specialist palliative care in Western Australia- and who misses out. *Palliative Medicine, 20*, p 439-445

96 AIHW. Residential aged care in Australia 2004-05: a statistical overview. Canberra: 2006.

97 Tuckett et al. (2014). What general practitioners said about the palliative care case conference in residential aged care: An Australian perspective. Part 1. *Progress in Palliative Care*, 22:2. 61-68.

98 Department of Health. Aged Care Funding Instrument; User Guide.

99 Dwyer, R., Gabbe, B., Stoelwinder, J., & Lowthian, J. (2014). A systematic review of outcomes following emergency transfer to hospital for residents of aged care facilities. *Age and Ageing*, 43: 759-766.

100 Dwyer, R., Gabbe, B., Stoelwinder, J., & Lowthian, J. (2014). A systematic review of outcomes following emergency transfer to hospital for residents of aged care facilities. *Age and Ageing*, 43: 759-766.

101 Dwyer, R., Gabbe, B., Stoelwinder, J., & Lowthian, J. (2014). A systematic review of outcomes following emergency transfer to hospital for residents of aged care facilities. *Age and Ageing*, 43: 759-766.

102 Van den Block, L., et al. (2007). Hospitalisations at the end of life: using a sentinel surveillance network to study hospital use and associated patient, disease and healthcare factors. BMC Health Services Research, 7:69.

103 Van den Block, L., et al. (2007). Hospitalisations at the end of life: using a sentinel surveillance network to study hospital use and associated patient, disease and healthcare factors. BMC Health Services Research, 7:69.

104 COSA and CVA Submission: Palliative Care in Australia. 2012.

105 Langton, J.M et al. (2016). Health service use and costs in the last 6 months of life in elderly decedents with a history of cancer: a comprehensive analysis from a health payer perspective. *British Journal of Cancer,* 114(11): 1293–130.

106 Brumlet, R.D., Enguidanos, S., & Cherin, D.A. (2003). Effectiveness of a home-based palliative care program for end of life. *Journal of Palliative Medicine,* 6(5), 715-24.

107 Smith, S., Brick, A., O'Hara, S., & Normand, C. (2013). Evidence on the cost and cost-effectiveness of palliative care: A literature review. *Palliative Medicine,* 28, p.130-150

108 Lewis JM, DiGiacomo M, Currow DC & Davidson PM 2011. Dying in the margins: understanding palliative care and socioeconomic deprivation in the developed world. *Journal of Pain and Symptom Management* 42:105–118Wood DJ, Clark D & Gatrell AC 2004. Equity of access to adult hospice inpatient care within north-west England. *Palliative Medicine* 18:543–549;

109 AIHW. Australis Welfare 2015; Growing older

110 Swerissen, H and Duckett, S. (2014) Dying Well. Grattan Institute

111 NSW Auditor-General's Report to Parliament. (2017). Planning and evaluating palliative care services in NSW

112 Huong Canh Le, B &Watt, J. (2010). Care of the dying in Australia's busiest hospital: benefits of palliative care consultation and methods to enhance access. *Journal of Palliative Medicine.* 13(7): 855-860

113 Parliament of Australia. The federal funding of palliative care in Australia.

114 NSW Auditor-General's Report to Parliament. (2017). Planning and evaluating palliative care services in NSW

115 Addington-Hall,J., Fakhoury, W., McCarthy, m. (1998). Specialist palliative care in non-malignant disease. *Palliative Medicine,* 12(6).

116 Duckett, S. & Willcox, S. (2015). The Australian Health Care System, 5th ed. Oxford university press; Melbourne

117 Parliament of Australia. The federal funding of palliative care in Australia.

118 AIHW. (2017). Palliative care services in Australia

119 Access Economics (2015). The economic value of informal care in Australia in 2015

120 Palliative Care in Victoria. The Facts

121 https://daughterlycare.com.au/what-does-private-in-home-care-cost

122 AIHW. (2017). Palliative care services in Australia

123 Department of Health. 2016. Medical Training Review Panel 19th Report

124 http://www.aihw.gov.au/workforce/medical/types-of-medical-practitioners/

125 AIHW. (2017). Palliative care services in Australia

126 Chiu, N. et al. (2015). Inadequacy of Palliative Training in the Medical School Curriculum, J Cancer Education, 30(4):749-53.

127 Urbis. (2017). Evaluation of the national palliative care strategy 2010 final report.

128 White, B., et al. (2014) Prevalence and predictors of advance directives in Australia. *Internal Medicine Journal.* 44(10), pp. 975-980.

129 White, B., et al. (2014) Prevalence and predictors of advance directives in Australia. *Internal Medicine Journal.* 44(10), pp. 975-980.

130 Bezzina, A.J. (2009). Prevalence of advance care directives in aged care facilities of the Northern Illawarra. *Emerg Med Australasi*a ;21:379–85.

131 Rhee, J., Zwar, N., & Kemp, L. (2012). Uptake and implementation of Advance Care Planning in Australia: findings of key informant interviews. *Australian Health Review,* 36, 98-104.

132 NSW Auditor-General's Report to Parliament. (2017). Planning and evaluating palliative care services in NSW

133 NSW government. 2016. NSW Government Commissioning and Contestability Practice Guide.

135 http://www.abc.net.au/news/2016-05-17/we-need-to-talk-about-death-more-senior-doctors-say/7422962

136 Le, B. et al. (2017). Palliative care in general practice: GP integration in caring for patients with advanced cancer. *Australian Family Physician*, 46, p.51-55.

137 Epstein, A.S., Prigerson, H.G., O'Reilly, E.M., & Maciewjewski, P.K. (2016). Discussions of life expectancy and changes in illness understanding in patients with advanced cancer. *Journal of Clinical Oncology*, 34(20).

138 Berwick, D.M. (2016). Era 3 for medicine and health care. *JAMA*, 315(13).

Chapter 6

Towards a More Competitive Medicare[*]

David Gadiel

"The increases in Commonwealth benefits, which came into
force on 1 January 1960, did not bring about any reduction
in the share of the total costs met by contributors [of health
funds]—for doctors raised their fees ...."

So wrote T H Kewley in 1965 of the 1959 Amendment to the National
Health Act 1953 that introduced Commonwealth benefit increases of up
to 100% for some 140 services.[1] In the quest of public policy to introduce
greater certainty to amounts that patients may pay to meet the cost of their
medical services, little has changed in the past 50 years.

Since at least the 1960s, the issue of medical fees and charges has been a
matter of controversy. Supported by public funding, doctors have remained
committed to fixing fees that suit themselves. The complicated and erratic
history of the way federal governments have attempted to restrict doctor
remuneration in Australia has yielded no success in either controlling
or influencing what they charge or what patients face in out-of-pocket
payments for the cost of their care. Nor have federal governments had
any success attempting to mandate cost-sharing for Medicare-funded
services—as exemplified by the eventual withdrawal of the Abbott
Government's 2014 GP co-payment policy.[2]

---

[*] First published as Towards a more competitive Medicare: The case for deregulating medical fees and
co-payments in Australia, Research Report 1, (Sydney: The Centre for Independent Studies, 2015).

Lack of ability to set with certainty what doctors charge and what patients pay in all circumstances has long remained a source of political embarrassment, because successive federal governments have promised what they have never had the power to deliver. Under the Australian Constitution, the federal government has no authority to regulate medical fees, and doctors have always had the power to set their own fees.

This chapter proposes a case for abolishing the Medicare Schedule Fee in light of its failure to establish a cooperative platform for dealings with the profession over the setting of fees. Well-intentioned interference in medical services pricing has contributed to supply conditions that are far from competitive; and (in spite of growth in publicly subsidised GP bulk billing) has not fulfilled the promise of universally equitable criteria for patient cost-sharing or service access. Given a specified Medicare benefit payable, each of these failings is best resolved in a market free of government interference.

History: The Schedule Fee, Medicare and bulk billing

The origin of the attempt to regulate medical fees —and provide equity of access to necessary medical services— dates from the spirit of co-operation that developed briefly between the federal government and the medical profession following introduction under the National Health Scheme of the 'most common fee' in 1970. Electoral demands for action to limit out-of-pocket charges for health care led the Commonwealth to rely on publishing a Schedule Fee in the Schedule of Medicare Benefits to influence what doctors may charge and to limit the size of the 'gap' paid by patients. Marked at first by a series of 'gentlemen's agreements', these efforts owe their origin to legislation introduced by the Gorton Coalition government in July 1970 that introduced what became known as 'the most common fee', later to become the Schedule Fee.

Subsequently, medical benefits were established with reference to the common fee list published by the Australian Medical Association (AMA). This represents the origin of the AMA's annual recommended fee list, now simply known as the AMA Fee List,[3] which is indexed for cost and wage increases.[4]

The Gorton government published its version of the list as the Schedule Fee, in fulfilment of an agreement it had negotiated with the AMA that doctors would accept the Schedule Fee to cover all but a small, set proportion of the cost of GP and other medical services paid for directly by patients.

Under the Gorton scheme, a patient was required to meet 80 cents of the cost of a standard GP consultation; for more expensive services or combinations of services, the patient contribution increased but was limited to $5.00 regardless of cost. Differential benefits were struck for some 300 medical services, to be reviewed biennially. For the first time, there was Commonwealth acknowledgement of a demarcation between the work of GPs and specialists; and this led to a distinction between the fees for GPs and specialists.

Even though the AMA agreed to encourage its members to observe common fees, there was no legal obligation under the legislation for doctors to abide by them, since government possessed no constitutional authority to control doctors' fees.

Notwithstanding the 'gentleman's agreement' to abide by the Schedule Fee, by February 1971, the AMA was recommending a unilateral fee increase to apply from February 1971—a harbinger of many to follow that fractured the nexūs between what doctors' actually charged, the AMA Fee List and the government's Schedule Fee.

Fee discontent continued to simmer throughout the 1970s, fuelled by disturbances to relativities that the Gorton common fee legislation had created between fees of GPs and specialists.

It gave specialists significantly greater market power than GPs. The realisation by specialists that they could command more than other members of their profession rankled with GPs and fuelled specialist fee aspirations.

The implementation of Medicare in October 1984 formalised a relationship whereby a Medicare benefit became payable at 85% of the Schedule Fee as prescribed in the Medicare Benefits Schedule (later 100% for GP services). Following the Canadian model, so-called bulk billing enabled patients to assign their Medicare benefit to doctors in full settlement of their liability and for Medicare to pay doctors directly. Doctors at the outset feared that as bulk billing became more widespread, the government-set rebate would effectively become their fee, as perhaps originally intended under the Gorton scheme and as eventually came to pass in the case of GPs in January 2005. This uncertainty created a source of continuing tension between government and doctors that was exemplified by the NSW doctors' dispute during the 1980s precipitated by the Hawke government's ill-fated attempt to regulate specialists' fees.

Preparatory to the implementation of Medicare in 1984, the Commonwealth offered the states untied hospital money on condition that the states persuaded doctors to sign contracts that would control costs and private practice in public hospitals. Doctors recognised this ploy for what it was: an attempt to use Commonwealth-State Medicare Agreements on hospital funding to circumvent the constitutional limitations on the power of government to control their fees.

The NSW Labor government took the lead in implementing the Commonwealth's bidding, with gazettal of an amendment to the Public Hospitals Act on 26 March 1983. This gave the NSW Health Minister power to make regulations on the appointment, management and control of visiting practitioners in public hospitals. Regulation 54(a) in particular made the appointment of Visiting Medical Officers (VMO) conditional on their not charging more than the Schedule Fee. The NSW dispute effectively became a proxy war for a national one over the power to control doctors' fees. The upshot was a costly and lengthy dispute involving the mass resignation of doctors from the NSW public hospital system. In September 1984, with the Commonwealth's agreement, the NSW government was obliged to capitulate and rescind Regulation 54(a).[5]

Any vestige of government's power to control doctors' fees was finally extinguished. The NSW doctors' dispute left no doubt that attempts to enforce the Schedule Fee as a statutory fee could risk igniting industrial anarchy, in recognition that under the Australian Constitution the government lacks power to control doctors' fees.[6] Recent High Court cases have affirmed that while government possesses constitutional power to regulate the manner in which medical services are provided, it lacks authority to use Medicare as a control on fees.[7]

What has now become the Medicare Schedule Fee thus imposes no obligations upon doctors: it remains simply a 'fee for benefit purposes'.[8] Hence government has resorted to incentive payments to pressure various types of billing practices to accommodate different policies of the day, using the Schedule Fee as a reference point.

Despite the equity and service access criteria underlining the declared intention of Medicare, government has been wary, since the debacle in NSW of 1984, of the market power of specialists and therefore loath to interfere with their billing practices. Instead it has oscillated between diametrically opposed policies to influence GP billing practices.

On the one hand, government has courted electoral popularity by seeking to augment the consumption of GP services. By contrast, both the Hawke Labor and Abbott Coalition governments have attempted to make patients more sensitive to the cost of care and to contain its financial burden to government by seeking to mandate a statutory GP co-payment.

The former goal was the motive behind the so-called Medicare Plus program introduced in 2003, whereby so as to minimise the likelihood of Concession card holders and patients under 16 incurring any gap between rebates and fees, GPs were paid a financial incentive to accept 85% of the Schedule Fee for services bulk billed to these patients. In January 2005 under the Strengthening Medicare program, GPs were further rewarded by being paid an incentive to accept 100% of the Schedule Fee for services they bulk billed.

These incentive payments are currently set within the range of $7.20 and $10.85 per service (depending on location and type of patient). Their impact (in conjunction with an increase in the GP workforce during the first decade of the century) has been to steadily drive the proportion of GP Medicare services bulk billed from 65.7% in 2003 to 85.2%% in the June quarter of 2017.[9] Between 2005 and 2016 Medicare expenditure on incentive payments (Medicare items 10990 and 10991) encouraging GPs to bulk bill at 100% of the Schedule Fee accordingly rose in nominal terms from $337 million to $603 million.[10] Bulk billing incentive payments are currently running at about 8.5% of all benefits attracted by the services of GPs.

Even though bulk billing incentives may cause the majority of GP services to be delivered at zero cost, significant welfare issues may be at stake for the minority who pay in excess of the Schedule Fee. This in turn brings into play the importance of creating greater all-round competitiveness in the supply of all medical services. Removal of extraneous price signals such as the Schedule Fee could make a significant contribution to competition reform. In pockets where lack of competition prevails, any type of public price signal can become a touchstone for excessive charging behaviour by GPs with market power, as well as by most specialists, that can cause significant social costs.

Co-payments versus bulk billing

In a bid to make patients more sensitive to the cost of care, and to contain the financial burden to government by inhibiting the demand for discretionary or unnecessary primary medical services for treating minor problems amenable to self-care or homeostasis, the Commonwealth on different occasions has sought to introduce a co-payment.

In 1991, a Labor administration introduced a $2.50 co-payment for GP services[11] that was revoked after three months, following a change of Prime Minister; and again in 2014 there was an unlegislated Budget measure that included encouraging GPs to collect a $7.00 co-payment with a $5.00 reduction in the Schedule Fee in conjunction with a 'low gap' incentive reward payment (in lieu of one for bulk billing).[12] This initiative and its watered down variations failed to gain Senate approval and at the time of writing had been abandoned[13], pending negotiations with the stakeholders.[14]

There is plainly an inconsistency in government paying GPs an incentive to bulk bill (or to adhere to any form of prescriptive low cost charging) at the same time as variously attempting a transition into partial measures of patient cost sharing. Even as the inconsistency in public policy remains unresolved, doctors' attitudes towards fees and cost sharing have been as equivocal as the government policy has been inconsistent. GPs have been willing to accept the government's bulk billing incentive payments, but—where conditions permit—they have been comfortable to charge patients what the market will bear. Specialists have generally opposed bulk billing, except (in some instances) for Concession Card holders.

A majority of GPs has embraced the Commonwealth's bulk billing incentive, and this has been conducive in turn to adoption of the Medicare benefit payable at 100% of the Schedule Fee as the benchmark for pricing most of their services. On the other hand, where lack of competitive conditions permit, GPs have been comfortable to charge what the market will bear— often in rural locations or in premium, high income metropolitan localities.[15] Practices in the Hunter area of NSW are an example of where most GPs routinely charge non-Concessional patients a co-payment of at least $30 for a standard consultation.[16] Some GP practices are now even charging a practice enrolment fee in addition to fees that exceed the Schedule Fee. Specialists have generally opposed bulk billing, except for some Concession card holders.

As Box 10 illustrates, there is a presumption under the status quo that diversity in local market conditions for GP services is likely contributing to a net welfare burden. Because it is unequally distributed within the population of GP primary care users, this burden constitutes a deadweight welfare loss of twin opposing dimensions: likely excessive use of care where it is 'free' (sometimes referred to as being indicative of 'supplier induced demand'[20]), in conjunction with the risk of underutilisation where patients incur uncompetitive prices associated with high doctor charges.[21] Where care is 'free' the extent of the distortion may be exacerbated by government bulk billing incentives.

Box 10: The welfare burden differential GP charging

- Distance between GP practices is significantly negatively associated with the proportion of patients who are bulk billed, and positively associated with the average price paid by patients who are not bulk billed as well as with the average price paid by all patients.[17] Because demand for GP services, relative to specialist services (at least), is price elastic (with a coefficient of -0.022),[18] it follows that concentration in undifferentiated service availability, potentiated by bulk billing incentives, increases the likelihood of the bulk billing price constituting a GP service floor price. Some GP services in areas of concentrated availability may command premiums for special skills or professional reputational considerations.

- The 'satisfaction' of the majority of Australians who live within relative proximity of a GP practice and who consume at a zero price (whether or not they are Concession cardholders) needs to be qualified by the likelihood of their service use being greater than necessary (since their demand becomes infinitely elastic at zero price).

- By contrast, as travel times increase, falls in the quantity of services consumed would be commensurate, inter alia, with the probability of fees charged by GPs exceeding the benefit. Moreover, the associated welfare loss could not necessarily be regarded as compensated by the 'satisfaction' of the majority who may pay less or not at all for their GP care (i.e. their capacity as gainers to 'bribe' losers). Their welfare loss, represented by an erosion of consumer surplus given by a Harberger triangle,[19] can be quantified in money terms (as 0.5 × $ value of services delivered × elasticity coefficient × the square of the relative price increase).

- Any loss so quantified would exclude any person not using GP services by virtue of being 'frozen out' of the market because of monopolistic pricing, excessive travel costs or both—and hence underestimate the extent of the actual loss. The estimate would also exclude the indirect loss of welfare arising from the value of the burden of any preventable illness that those afflicted would be 'willing to pay' to avoid.

Market distortions occur because doctors are rational market players. They are conscious that in localities with an abundant supply of GPs or with ready access to hospital outpatient services that may substitute for primary GP care, the overall revenue accruing from the incremental financial gain of government bulk billing incentive payments in conjunction with revenue collected from their charges 'held' at the Schedule Fee will exceed the financial reward from setting fees above the Schedule. These GPs are content to forgo the prospect of the higher margins available from above Schedule Fee charges (at perhaps lower service volumes) and to settle for delivering larger volumes of patient throughput associated with 100% Schedule Fee bulk billing—possibly to the extent of excess. This has potential to constitute a social harm associated with inefficiency, with budgetary implications that the government's cost sharing initiatives have sought to address.

On the other hand, in localities less well endowed with primary medical care, far from anchoring the benefit payable, the Schedule Fee has constituted a springboard that could offer incentives for GPs to sacrifice some bulk billing incentive rewards and rather to maximise rent seeking behaviour for which customers (including even some Concession card holders) may be obliged to pay. The premiums that GP services attract where they, or services of outpatient substitute services, are in short supply are analogous to the premiums that most specialist services (also in short supply) command in excess of the Schedule Fee.[22]

Hence the contradiction evident between the AMA's outspoken opposition to iniquities alleged of the proposed 2014 co-payment for GP services,[23] and its silence in the face of rural GP billing practices or specialist charges that— respectively depending upon the locality of their practice or the discipline of their specialism or both—may exceed the Schedule Fee by a factor of many times.[24]

Fear of losing custom—due to the disincentive price effect of a GP co-payment or any form of cost sharing in localities with heavy concentrations of doctors—has readily masqueraded as an argument against risking loss of access to GP preventive health services; and thereby allegedly increasing the exposure of government to downstream costs, and patients to the burden of avoidable hospitalisations and chronic disease.

The AMA has accordingly described the more recent version of the government's co-payment as a "wrecking ball".[25] Public health enthusiasts allied with the public health lobby have made common cause with the GPs who oppose the 2014 co-payment.[26]

Officially the AMA, never an advocate of bulk billing, has long distanced itself from the adequacy of the Schedule Fee. Its own Fee List covering all areas of medical practice (and intended to be confidential to AMA members) is substantially higher. In the case of a GP standard Level B consultation (MBS Item 23), for instance, the AMA at the time of writing listed a fee of $78.00[27] compared with a fee of $37.05 in the Medicare Schedule. It is hard to reconcile the AMA's inflated fee list with its public disavowal of the relatively small GP co-payment proposed in the 2014 Budget, which the AMA opposed on social equity criteria.

The AMA's official position is that GPs, as in the case of all doctors, may be obliged to charge increasing patient out-of-pocket costs to avoid erosion of their incomes or deterioration in the quality of the service they provide or both, because of intermittent freezes of the Schedule Fee and the reluctance of government to adhere to fee indexation.[28] The AMA thus encourages doctors to charge a 'fair and reasonable fee' having regard to their practice costs.[29]

Gap cover for out-of-pocket costs

Some private health insurers seem ready to accommodate doctors who adopt charging practices that pass on to patients what the doctors may consider their unrequited costs. Medibank Private, for instance, is trialling a private insurance model that intersects public Medicare coverage of GP primary care. For persons covered on its hospital tables, Medibank Private's trial is designed to guarantee 'priority' access to out-of-hospital GP services at zero price in south east Queensland at Independent Practitioner Network (IPN) practices owned by Sonic Health Limited. If widely adopted, it would have the potential to neutralise the impact of any government attempts to encourage the implementation of GP cost sharing.[30]

Besides representing a likely infringement of s126 of the Health Insurance Act 1973 (which seeks to prevent private health insurers writing cover for out-of-hospital medical services attracting a Medicare benefit),[31] it remains to be seen whether medical gap cover inherent in the Medibank Private trial will further its stated objective of intercepting otherwise undetectable health problems that will keep patients out of hospital. If hospital drawing rates remain the same, ultimately such a model—although doubtless popular with some doctors[32]—could result in health insurance premium increases due to incremental medical costs that could not be debited to the Reinsurance Trust Fund (a risk equalisation scheme to prevent destabilisation of the health insurance industry) and would test the willingness of Medibank Private's contributors to pay for a dubious benefit.

During the lead in to Medibank Private's Initial public offering the Minister for Health did not seek a judgement to test the validity of its trial under the Act—very likely for good commercial reasons. Unhappily, this could open the door to other health funds in partnership with competing medical chains with an appetite for market share to emulate Medibank Private's model.[33]

Analogous to the Medibank Private trial—and contradicting the principle of cost sharing in a like manner—are no-gap service contracts that health funds have negotiated with hospitals and specialists. Since 1 July 1995 the federal government has permitted health funds to offer no-gap or known-gap private hospital insurance covering inpatient medical services in excess of the statutory 25% inpatient medical benefit payable on their Basic tables and linked to the Schedule Fee (although gaps for some hospital charges may still apply).

Subject to any applicable deductibles, these private hospital tables remove or reduce the risk to private inpatients of a liability for medical cost sharing. No-gap entitlements are available to patients if they use doctors who have entered into Medical Purchaser Provider Agreements with their health fund, provided that fees for their Medicare services, although exceeding Schedule Fees, do not exceed fee for gap limits the fund has set. Funds then pay the difference between the agreed no-gap fee and the Basic 75% Medicare inpatient rebate.

Not all doctors participate in such no-gap arrangements, in which case a fund may pay an extra benefit, provided that the doctor beforehand advises the patient in writing of the gap they will face and obtains their informed financial consent. The higher benefit payable for such a known-gap will then limit the patient's liability to a prescribed maximum for each Medicare item (typically $400 per item). Indeed, the AMA believes it is quite reasonable for privately insured patients to meet the cost of gaps for specialist treatment for cancer and the like if fees exceed the available gap cover.[34]

During the quarter ending September 2017, medical services paid for by health funds under no-gap and known-gap arrangements averaged 145% of the Schedule Fee. These excess fees covered 88% of inpatient hospital medical services that were provided to patients under no-gap arrangements and 7% provided under known-gaps.[35]

Although these gap arrangements target the services of specialists—and do not directly impinge on the government's declared policy of GP co-payments (as in the case of Medibank Private's GP trial and government 100% Schedule Fee incentive)—they analogously reduce the transparency to patients of fees raised by doctors and run contrary to cost sharing principles designed to evoke consumer price consciousness.

Impact of gap cover on fee setting

Allowing health funds to write no-gap or known-gap cover for private inpatient specialist care underwritten by private hospital insurance tables has compounded the inconsistencies that abound in government policy.

Since demand for specialist services is likely to be considerably more price inelastic than for primary care, rather than offering insured patients enhanced access to services—as they would in any case have used them because of necessity—the main impact of no-gap or known-gap inpatient extra medical coverage is to embolden doctors to introduce further increases in their fees. The attempt to maintain or to extend no-gap cover margins, cascading from a benchmark such as the Schedule Fee thus becomes self-defeating.

Since demand for specialist services is likely to be considerably more price inelastic than demand for GP primary care where it is abundant or where there is substitute hospital outpatient care,[36] rather than giving privately insured patients enhanced access to specialist services—as patients would in any case have used them because of their necessity—the main impact of gap inpatient extra medical coverage is simply to create a vortex for specialist fee increases.

As health funds from time to time increase the level of the available gap benefit to compensate for such higher fees, doctors become emboldened to introduce further increases in their fees for inpatient services, and the attempt to maintain or to extend full gap cover becomes self-defeating.[37]

No-gap and known-gap insurance cover has consequently had a material impact on the cost of health insurance.[38] During the early years of gap cover's rapid uptake (2002-04), its share of hospital benefits paid by health funds per single equivalent contributor rose at an annual rate of 17.7% compared to 7% for hospital accommodation benefits.[39] With prostheses, payments for specialist services have thus been a significant factor in the increasing benefit cost of private hospital tables.

No-gap arrangements have contributed to cycles of increases in contributions payable, causing those tables to become less attractive to low risk contributors who may be encouraged to migrate to lower tables or to relinquish their cover.

To the extent that the associated costs of such incremental benefits are debited to the Reinsurance Trust Fund, it contributes to the overall costs of health insurance over which, because of their lack of power to bargain with doctors, health insurers have little control.[40]

While the Schedule Fee provides the benchmark for a statutory inpatient Medicare benefit of 25% for private patients (rather than Medicare's 15% for out-of-hospital care), it also acts as a baseline for underpinning the scope of the margin available to funds (associated with actual specialist charges) to compete destructively with each other in their no-gap and known-gap private hospital insurance offerings. The continuing upward pressure on health insurance premiums that results has progressively adverse cost consequences, which are often referred to as a 'death spiral of adverse selection'.[41]

BUPA (Australia's second largest health insurer) goes so far as to argue a case for extending no-gap inpatient cover by further deregulating the private health insurance industry to permit no-gap cover for out-of-hospital specialist services. It claims this would "be consistent with transparency of costs ... (and) inform consumers and improve competition" by delivering "a complete out-of-pocket experience for members for entire episodes of care".[42]

By shielding patients from the price effects of specialist charging behaviour, BUPA's agenda nevertheless appears less to do with transparency than with underwriting specialists' billing practices and stifling price competition between them. It would compound the problems of no-gap inpatient cover and once again contradict government's cost sharing agenda. To the extent that if such no-gap cover were ever incorporated in hospital tables, taxpayers would also pay more via the private health insurance subsidy.

The anti-competitive effect of the Schedule Fee

There are many imperfections in the market for medical services in Australia's fee for service environment, including considerable scope for GPs and specialists to set their prices, depending on their geographical location and their area of specialisation.[43] Aside from rigid demarcations that exist in the labour market for health services and entry barriers to establishing a career in medicine, an underlying contributory factor is the publication of the Medicare Schedule Fee.

It is paradoxical that government should go to the trouble of setting a fee for Medicare services, when it has no constitutional authority or power to control fees. The reality is that government strategies to impose either statutory co-payments or to introduce any charging conformity based on the Schedule Fee are as limited in 2015 as they were in the 1960s, yet the fiction persists that the existence of the Schedule Fee contributes in some way to public policy.

The hierarchy of doctors' fees not paid by government—whether in the nature of a GP co-payment, charges above the Medicare benefit for any other private medical services, or the margin by which medical fees for private inpatient care exceed the threshold set by the Basic inpatient medical rebate—ultimately derives from formal acknowledgement of the vestigial Schedule Fee in the Health Insurance Act 1973.

A climate of expectation ensues whereby the Schedule Fee becomes the first rung in the hierarchy: it is useful to government to help anchor higher GP charges through bulk billing incentives; and it can also act as a general spur for any doctors with sufficient market power to calibrate additional tiers of charging according to local market conditions, having regard as well to the AMA Fee list—with the destabilising corollary, in the case of private inpatient care, of driving the amount of available gap cover increasingly higher in a continuing upward spiral.

Besides their direct burden upon consumers, doctor charges based on market power are costly (via higher premiums) to households contributing to higher private hospital tables. They also have an impact on state governments meeting the cost of contractual VMO work in public systems (via either individual employment contracts or other agreements).

The competitive effect of abolishing the Schedule Fee

Medicare arrangements should match the constitutional realities. GPs charge the way they are rewarded to charge. The government should save itself the contradiction and the cost of paying GPs incentives to bulk bill while trying to advocate the virtue of patients becoming accountable for at least some of the cost of their care.

The Schedule Fee should be abolished hand-in-hand with abolition of GP bulk billing incentive payments for which GPs received a government subsidy of some $0.6 billion in 2016. Abolition of the Schedule Fee (by setting it at zero) in conjunction with its GP incentives would create an arm's length between fees actually charged and benefits that could be claimed. Without the distortion of a billing incentive attached to an official price signal, GP charges would gradually find their own level, but not necessarily linked to the Medicare benefit—as indeed would tend to occur for all doctor charges. Instead, government could simply publish a standalone benefit payable on items listed on the Medicare Benefits Schedule. The notion of quasi-statutory co-payments would then fall away and save governments the political embarrassment of trying to introduce them. This change could be accomplished under the Health Insurance Regulations without legislative affirmation.

Individual doctors would retain freedom to set their own fees as they saw fit according to local market conditions. Their correctly itemised services would continue to attract Medicare benefits. Those GPs with concerns about co-payments creating a barrier to their patients' accessing primary preventive health services would remain at liberty to set their fees at the Medicare benefit and to absorb the loss of the bulk billing reward payment on their own account.

In the case of specialists, abolition of the Schedule Fee would undermine the baseline that accommodates differential gap and no-gap private insurance for inpatient services and help create thereby opportunities for a more competitive repricing of specialist services.

GPs with market power, and most specialists, who are accustomed to charging fees exceeding the benefit, would remain free to compete in the market place but without the Schedule Fee as a background price signal or as a benchmark for Basic inpatient medical benefits (which insurance funds would competitively determine without government regulation). In the case of GPs, individual doctors (if they felt it necessary) would have the inherent capacity to privately recoup, to the extent possible in the free market, the equivalent of the GP billing incentive subsidy they had lost.

Under a simplified and reformed Medicare, co-payments (and the public odium they clearly attract) would hence nevertheless become the business of doctors rather than of governments. This would focus health consumers' minds on what doctors charge instead of what government pays, and would engineer a shift towards greater competitiveness in setting medical fees—as in markets for medical services in countries without price signals, such as New Zealand and Singapore.

GPs could continue to accept assigned benefits and charge patients for any residual privately determined 'out-of-pocket costs' that prevailed—although it is likely that legislation would be required to permit a benefit to be assigned if gaps charged exceeded the amount of the assignment. If legislative change proved a barrier, alternative administrative arrangements for paying benefits could be adopted, such as those currently used for specialists whereby patients pay in full, with the doctor's practice simultaneously claiming a benefit on behalf of the patient through a Medicare EFTPOS link and directly crediting the patient's benefit to their bank account. In any event, the inherent driver of medical fees in most situations would be a shift towards greater competitiveness and a distancing of government from fee setting arrangements.

Of course, removal of the bulk billing subsidy may not be popular with GPs. They cannot, however, have it both ways. It will always remain their prerogative to advocate for remuneration exceeding the benefit to compensate their loss of incentive payments. But rather than continuing to shift their business risk on to third parties, they should wear this risk by testing the market for themselves as any other small businesses are bound to do, without the umbrella of public patronage. The incentive was, after all, first introduced quite suddenly as an outright windfall to GPs without regard to scope either for congruent productivity gain or for the attainment of new standards of quality assurance.

Abolition of the Schedule Fee would have systemic implications not just for GP co-payments. Its abolition would have ramifications, for instance, for operation of indexed Medicare Safety Net thresholds.[44] These are designed to provide relief for individuals and families with 'unusually' high out-of-pocket out-of-hospital medical services costs. The 2017 baseline (or 'Original') Threshold provides 100% of Schedule Fee cover for out-of-hospital medical services once the sum of the series of a person's gap payments to doctors exceeding the Schedule Fee reaches $453.20 in a calendar year.[45] Formalisation of such gaps by way of the Schedule Fee creates further avenues mainly for specialists to raise their fees above the Schedule Fee and defeats the purpose of the Safety Net.

Extended Medicare Safety Nets (EMSN) rely on higher thresholds and refund 80% of all out-of-pocket costs for out-of-hospital Medicare services above the threshold in a calendar year—$656.30 for Concession card holders and $2,056.30 for the general population for 2017.[46] EMSNs create a further layer of subsidy to accommodate what are often prohibitive specialist out-of-hospital charging practices. A 2009 study found that because the EMSN simply targeted a doctor's bill, nearly 80% of its cost went towards higher specialist fees.[47] The competition effect of removing the Schedule Fee would reduce the need for all routine Safety Nets. If instead the government were to introduce a modified and carefully targeted Safety Net to cover for chronic and catastrophic health events affecting the poor, it would reduce at least the extent of its moral hazard exposure.

Although Australia is not the only country to publish an official fee list for medical services, some countries recognise fee lists as potentially anti-competitive. In Singapore, a country with health outcomes comparable with Australia, doctors charge patients without reference either to fee lists or indeed to any list of service definitions. Free market pricing of medical services in Singapore not only plays a role in encouraging health consumers to make discriminating choices; it also constitutes an incentive for practitioners to keep their costs down and to maintain affordable charging practices within the means of patients.[48] The market for medical services in New Zealand bears more resemblance to Australia's than to Singapore's. GPs are contractors to New Zealand's public health system but they independently set the fees they collect from patients over and above their public remuneration without reference to government or other fee lists.[49]

Even if Australia were to abolish its Schedule Fee, the move to a free market for medical services under Medicare in Australia would be constrained by the continued existence of the list of Medicare item numbers; defining the services for which a benefit was payable, and the restrictions applying to their use. This would thwart scope for competition in new product service offerings. The main competitive driver would be price competition centred upon Medicare service definitions with a capacity to charge fees ranging between the benefit payable and various levels above, depending upon local market conditions, doctors' respective skill sets and their special interests and professional reputations.

This would nevertheless at least create greater opportunities for doctors to more aggressively advertise their fees and to create greater price transparency as occurs in the case of dentists and optical dispensers. It could encourage the adoption of voluntary peer review mechanisms (as sanctioned by antitrust authorities in the United States[50]) to handle complaints about doctor overcharging. It may also offer scope for GPs to offer their regular patients increased service content for the service definitions.

A further step in moving towards a more competitive Medicare would be to refine the definitions of Medicare item numbers so as to introduce greater flexibility in the service descriptions, including greater scope for blended payments and for care perhaps involving term contracts covering one or more item numbers.

AMA Fee List and competition policy

Abolition of the Schedule Fee, and as a corollary the related fee list maintained by the Department of Veterans Affairs, would serve to focus attention on the private medical price signals remaining in the market, and create a focus for their ultimate removal: the AMA Fee List and other derivative lists that the industrial wings of some specialist disciplines maintain, such as the Relative Value Guide of the Australian Society of Anaesthetists.[51] Although the AMA claims that its fees are "only a guide" and not recommended fees, it is clear that many doctors and medical practices (and procedural specialists in particular) overtly adopt confidential AMA list fees privately disclosed between themselves as their own. Practice web sites are legion allowing, for example, that "consultation fees are at the rate prescribed by AMA"; or that the doctor "bills at the recommended AMA fee"; or that fees "are guided by the AMA", etc.

Where competition is jeopardised through access issues or the risk of cartelisation because of professional entry barriers, the market becomes progressively receptive to extraneous price signals such as published (government or private) fee lists.

Although it is silent about doctor fee setting, the Competition Policy Review Draft Report (the Harper Review),[52] released on 22 September 2014, believes that "private disclosure of pricing information has the potential to harm consumer interests as it can facilitate collusion on coordination between competitors..."

As things stand, medical services are subject to competition policy, adjudicated by the ACCC, administering the Competition and Consumer Act 2010—previously the Trade Practices Act 1974 (TPA). Part IV of the TPA (dealing with restrictive trade practices) applied originally only to professionals working in incorporated business structures. The TPA did not affect doctors working as sole practitioners or in unincorporated partnerships. This may have represented some sort of implicit acknowledgment of a special relationship claimed to be inherent between doctors and patients, based on quality of service and ethical criteria. This changed in 1995 when, under the aegis of Council of Australian Governments (COAG), the states and territories enacted their respective Competition Policy Reform Acts, incorporating provisions of the TPA and extending its reference to "persons". In November 1995, the ACCC gave new guidance to various health stakeholders, including individual professionals and associations, advising them of issues such as fee setting and arrangements with other professionals that could put them at risk of contravening the law.[53]

Competition law in relation to the practice of medicine as it stands nevertheless remains anomalous. It is intended to prohibit competing doctors from collectively agreeing on the fees they will charge patients, or participating in agreements that claim to recommend prices but which in reality fix prices by agreement. However, since 2002 the ACCC has issued various authorisations, including consent to "capped fee structures"[54] as well as permission for doctors working in partnership in the same practice to discuss and agree fees. In 2013 the latter type of authorisation was extended to allow GPs practising in a partnership to collectively bargain with public hospitals for public medical services such as after-hours consultations.[55]

GPs working in associateships meeting certain criteria, including accreditation by The Royal Australian College of General Practitioners (RACGP), may also discuss and agree on fees;[56] but surgeons who work as associates evidently are regarded as practising as individuals and cannot discuss fees.[57] Moreover, in setting their fees, even though doctors may freely consult the AMA Fee List, they cannot legally discuss their fee policies with other doctors or partnerships.

Whilst there have been isolated cases where the ACCC has secured judgements against individual doctors,[58] it is evident that competition law as it relates to the pricing of medical services continues to be tested in a series of case-by-case authorisations or Federal Court judgements. This is far from satisfactory. Under the present law it appears challenging to disentangle price signalling and possible implicit collusion by way of the AMA Fee List from the act of consulting the List to arrive at a fee. An amendment of The Health Insurance Regulations to abolish the Schedule Fee hence remains a necessary but insufficient condition for a move toward competitive fee setting for medical services.

While in Australia the ACCC has never made any formal decision on the AMA Fee List, by contrast in 2007 the Singapore Medical Association (SMA) withdrew its Guideline of Fees (in force since 1987) to avoid the risk of contravening Singapore's Competition Act. In 2010, in recognition of the harm that fee recommendations can do to competition, the Competition Commission subsequently affirmed the SMA's action.[59] The Commission found that the Guideline infringed section 34 of the Competition Act by breaching prohibition of agreements that have as "their object ... restriction or distortion of competition within Singapore" and that the Guideline delivered no net economic benefit.

Making Medicare More Competitive

It is ironic that the AMA Fee List originated with the blessing of government for purposes of calculating the Schedule Fee and defining the content of the Medicare Benefits Schedule. Both became integral to the Health Insurance Act 1973. The public policy environment has since changed dramatically. High expectations that an AMA List would harmonise with a Schedule Fee on a gentlemen's agreement were quickly dashed. The nexus that existed between them was lost a year after it was forged and has never been re-established.

Where, due to lack of competition, doctors do not bulk bill, the Schedule Fee has the potential to encourage medical service pricing by some GPs and most specialists in a way quite the opposite of what was originally intended. Since it cannot control what doctors charge, the Schedule Fee has no intrinsic public policy worth in determining patient out-of-pocket payments—except in situations where, at much additional cost to government, doctors are paid to observe it. As a corollary, it therefore fails as an efficient anchor for any official co-payment policy; neither is it recognised by the AMA, because doctors are always free to set their charges in the manner of their choosing at or above the statutory benefit payable. Where doctors exert market power, the Schedule Fee becomes a baseline that brings an inflated AMA Fee List into play, inviting GPs and specialists alike to set fees that risk becoming a charge against consumer welfare.

The primary concern of funding agencies (government and health funds) should thus be the setting of benefits—and in the interests of efficiency, at levels that leave room for a more effective market, free of the burden of bulk billing subsidies or no-gap insurance, to arbitrate co-payments and out-of-pocket specialist charges. The Schedule Fee has become redundant: it has failed its original purpose and much more; and should accordingly be abolished to facilitate greater scrutiny of the effect of the AMA Fee List and permit more competitive market forces to play their part dispassionately in determining fairer fees.

Endnotes

1 T H Kewley Social Security in Australia 1900-72, Sydney University Press, 1973 (2nd Ed), p 363

2 Statement, The Hon Sussan Ley, Minister for Health, "Government continues Medicare consultation" 3 March 2015 http://www.health.gov.au/internet/ministers/publishing.nsf/Content/223AE2CC4BB4C324CA257DFD0014DDD3/$File/SL013.pdf

3 https://ama.com.au/ausmed/ama-list-medical-services-and-fees-18

4 AMA List of medical services and fees, 2012 http://www.amawa.com.au/wp-content/uploads/2013/03/fees-nov.pdf

5 The NSW doctors' dispute is chronicled in Australian Academy of Medicine and Surgery, History of Medicine, http://www.aams.org.au/contents.php?subdir=library/history/funding_prof_med_au/&filename=1983to1993; see also Peter Catts How to knife surgeons, the life and times of a crusading surgeon—a memoir, Healthy Lifestyle Publishing, Rhodes NSW, 2014, Chapters 14 - 18

6 Section 51(xxiiiA) of the Australian Constitution forbids any legislation that would have the effect of the 'civil conscription' of doctors.

7 Thomas Faunce "Constitutional limits on federal legislation practically compelling medical employment: Wong v Commonwealth; Selim v Professional Services Review Committee" Journal of Law and Medicine, 2009,17: 196-205 https://law.anu.edu.au/sites/all/files/users/u9705219/236-lawrep-017-jlm-jl-0196.pdf

8 Section 9 of the Health Insurance Act 1973 provides that Medicare benefits be calculated by reference to fees for medical services set out in Tables prescribed The Health Insurance Regulations.

9 Medicare quarterly statistics, Department of Human Services, http://www.health.gov.au/internet/main/publishing.nsf/Content/Quarterly-Medicare-Statistics

10 Department of Human Services, http://medicarestatistics.humanservices.gov.au/statistics/mbs_item.jsp

11 Medicare, The Changes to Medicare: once you've read the booklet it's all very simple, 1991, Canberra

12 Commonwealth of Australia, Budget 2014-15 Health, 13 May 2104

13 Latika Bourke "Abbott abandons plan to slash Medicare rebate for doctors' visits", Sydney Morning Herald, 15 January, 2015 http://www.smh.com.au/federal-politics/political-news/abbott-abandons-plan-to-slash-medicare-rebate-for-doctors-visits-20150115-12r447.htm

14 Statement, The Hon Sussan Ley, 3 March 2015 as above", with consequential re-numbering of footnotes that follow.

15 Hugh Gravelle et al, Competition prices and quality in the market for physician consultations, Melbourne Institute Working Paper 23/13, Melbourne Institute of Applied Economic and Social Research, University of Melbourne, June 2013 http://www.melbourneinstitute.com/downloads/working_paper_series/wp2013n23.pdf

16 Donna Page "Hunter doctors baulk at bulk billing", Newcastle Herald, 23 November, 2009 http://www.theherald.com.au/story/449049/hunter-doctors-baulk-at-bulk-billing/

17 Hugh Gravelle et al, as above

18 Hugh Gravelle et al, as above

19 Arnold C. Harberger "Monopoly and resource allocation" The American Economic Review, 1954, 64:2:77-88

20 Jeff Richardson "The inducement hypothesis: that doctors generate demand for their own services" in J. van der Gaag and M. Perlman (eds) Health, Economics and Health Economics, Contributions to Economic Analysis No 137, 1981, North Holland, Amsterdam

21 David Gadiel and Lee Ridoutt, The specialist medical workforce and specialist service provision in rural areas, Department of Human Services and Health and MWDRC No 1, AGPS, Canberra, 1995 http://trove.nla.gov.au/work/9818047?q&versionId=45878238

22 David Gadiel et al as above

23 AMA, "Beach report further evidence that proposed co-payments hurt the most vulnerable", 7th July, 2014, https://ama.com.au/media/beach-report-further-evidence-proposed-co-payments-hurt-most-vulnerable

24 Terry Barnes, "The AMA cannot claim moral high ground on co-payments" The Australian, 20 June 2014, http://www.theaustralian.com.au/opinion/ama-cannot-claim-moral-high-ground-on-copayments/story-e6frg6zo-1226960453661?login=1

25 Nick Pedley "GP co-payment: AMA says government's revised plan a wrecking ball" ABC News, 17th December, 2014 http://www.abc.net.au/news/2014-12-17/gp-co-payment-opposed-by-australian-medical-association/5974342

26 AMA, as above

27 https://ama.com.au/media/medicare-freeze-forcing-gp-fees

28 Access Economics (for the Australian Medical Association) Indexation of MBS rebates for GP consultation items, June 2004 https://ama.com.au/sites/default/files/documents/160604_Indexation_of_MBS_Rebates_FINAL.pdf

29 AMA, "Guide for patients on how the health care system funds medical care" Undated, http://scco.com.au/wp-content/uploads/2015/02/Guide-for-Patients-on-How-the-Health-Care-System-Funds-Medical-Care.pdf

30 Sean Parnell "Medibank Private to pick up GP costs in trial" The Australian, 10 January, 2014 http://www.theaustralian.com.au/national-affairs/policy/medibank-private-to-pick-up-gp-costs-in-trial/story-fn59nokw-1226798584183#

31 Section 126 of the Health Insurance Act 1973 prohibits private health insurance for medical services attracting a Medicare benefit, except for services that are hospital treatment or hospital-substitute treatment.

32 Whilst the AMA opposes statutory co-payments, curiously it has also opposed Medibank Private's gap cover trial. It alleges that it could constitute a threat in the form of "US-style managed care"; ABC 7.30 Report "AMA warns Government against US-style health system", 23 July 2014 http://www.abc.net.au/7.30/content/2014/s4052418.htm

33 David Gadiel "Integrating insurance with health service provision – a volatile partnership. Ideas, CIS, 24 October 2014 http://www.cis.org.au/publications/ideasthecentre/article/5347-integrating-insurance-with-health-service-provision-a-volatile-partnership

34 Sue Dunlevy "Patients happy to pay for cosmetic surgery should not complain about gap fees for cancer says AMA" Herald Sun, 12th November, 2014 http://m.heraldsun.com.au/news/national/patients-happy-to-pay-for-cosmetic-surgery-should-not-complain-about-gap-fees-for-cancer-says-ama/story-fni0xqrb-1227121031218?nk=8eedb3ff65fdca8bfcb90d7197d4f222

35 http://www.apra.gov.au/PHI/Publications/Documents/1711-QPHIS-20170930.pdf

36 Darrel P. Doessel The Economics of medical diagnosis: technological change and health expenditure, Avebury, Aldershot, 1992 http://bookdir.info/?p=531410; Private Health Insurance Administration Council Competition in the Australian private health insurance market, Research Paper 1, 3 June 2013, http://phiac.gov.au/wp-content/uploads/2013/12/PHIAC_Research_Paper_No1-new-format.pdf

37 Private Health Insurance Administration Council, as above

38 Private Health Insurance Administration Council, Operations of the Registered Benefit Organisations, Annual Report, 2002-03 http://phiac.gov.au/wp-content/uploads/2012/08/82pa2003.pdf

39 Andrew P Gale "What price health? Private health insurance cost pressures and product pricing" presented to the Institute of Actuaries of Australia 2005 Biennial Convention 8 May – 11 May 2005 http://actuaries.asn.au/Library/Events/Conventions/2005/1.c-Gale_Andrew_Final%20Paper_What%20Price%20Health_050419.PDF

40 John Menadue AO and Ian McCauley "Private health insurance: high in cost and low in equity, Centre for Policy Development, January 2012 http://www.ianmcauley.com/academic/cpd/phijan2012.pdf

41 Peter Zweifel and Roland Eisen (2012), Insurance economics, Springer, Heidelberg

42 Out-of-pocket costs in Australian healthcare, BUPA, Submission to Senate Standing Committees on Community Affairs, 21 May, 2014 http://www.google.com.au/url?sa=t&rct=j&q=&esrc=s&source=web&cd=2&ved=0C-CcQFjAB&url=http%3A%2F%2Fwww.aph.gov.au%2FDocumentStore.ashx%3Fid%3D-fa5dfe76-d06a-48ca-ac33-689a5a808143%26subld%3D252865&ei=XR3JU8vlG9H78QX-g0IDoDw&usg=AFQjCNErNfJthNdMGBxz_kCwAn6CoLQ2Ug&bvm=bv.71198958,d.dGc

43 Hugh Gravelle et al, as above

44 2014 Medicare Safety Net Thresholds http://www.humanservices.gov.au/customer/enablers/medicare/medicare-safety-net/medicare-safety-net-thresholds

45 Department of Health, Medicare Safety Net Thresholds from 1 January, 2015 http://www.health.gov.au/internet/mbsonline/publishing.nsf/Content/news-2014-10-07-latest-news-EMSNJan2015

46 http://www.mbsonline.gov.au/internet/mbsonline/publishing.nsf/Content/Factsheet-ExtendedMedicareSafetyNetThresholds-Jan2017

47 Elizabeth Savage et al, Extended Medicare Safety Net, Review Report 2009, A Report by the Centre for Health Economics Research and Evaluation, prepared for the Australian Government Department of Health and Ageing, 2009 http://www.health.gov.au/internet/main/publishing.nsf/Content/Review_%20Extended_Medicare_Safety_Net/$File/ExtendedMedicareSafetyNetReview.pdf

48 David Gadiel and Jeremy Sammut Lessons from Singapore: opt out health savings accounts for Australia, CIS, July 2014

49 Nicolas Timmins and Chris Ham, The quest for integrated health and social care. A case study in Canterbury, New Zealand, The King's Fund, London 2013 http://www.kingsfund.org.uk/sites/files/kf/field/field_publication_file/quest-integrated-care-new-zealand-timmins-ham-sept13.pdf

50 FTC advisory opinions in National Capital Society of Plastic and Reconstructive Surgeons, 23 April 1991

51 Relative Value Guide http://www.asa.org.au/UploadedDocuments/Publications/MEDIAPACKrvg.pdf

52 Commonwealth of Australia, The Australian Government Competition Policy Review, 22 September, 2014 http://competitionpolicyreview.gov.au/files/2014/09/Competition-policy-review-draft-report.pdfcy-review-draft-report.pdf

53 ACCC, A Guide to the Trade Practices Act for the Health Sector, November, 1995, Australian Government Publishing Company, Canberra

54 'ACCC proposes to authorise revised capped fees for the Canberra After Hours Locum Medical Service, October 2006; http://www.accc.gov.au/media-release/accc-proposes-to-authorise-revised-capped-fees-for-the-canberra-after-hours-locum

55 ACCC authorisation No A91334 https://www.mja.com.au/careers/198/9/price-right

56 'ACCC gives certainty to doctors within general practices on fee-setting' December 2002; http://www.accc.gov.au/media-release/accc-gives-certainty-to-doctors-within-general-practices-on-fee-setting

57 Ian Wheatley, Professional autonomy of Victorian surgeons in the context of law and ethics, Doctor of Philosophy Thesis, Deakin University, 2012, Chapter 3 https://dro.deakin.edu.au/eserv/DU:30048437/wheatley-professionalautomony-2012A.pdf

58 'Federal Court finds Rockhampton obstetricians' boycott of 'no gap' billing breached competition laws', October 2002, http://www.accc.gov.au/media-release/federal-court-finds-rockhampton-obstetricians-boycott-of-no-gap-billing-breached; 'ACCC files against Sydney anaesthetists, Society of Anaesthetists', October 1997, http://www.accc.gov.au/media-release/accc-files-against-sydney-anaesthetists-society-of-anaesthetists; 'Federal Court declares doctor attempted to induce boycotts of bulk-billing, after hours service at medical centre', March 2003, http://www.accc.gov.au/media-release/federal-court-declares-doctor-attempted-to-induce-boycotts-of-bulk-billing-after-hours; 'ACCC alleges price fixing at Joondalup Health Campus', July 2000, http://www.accc.gov.au/media-release/accc-alleges-price-fixing-at-joondalup-health-campus

59 Com http://competitionpolicyreview.gov.au/files/2014/09/Competition-policy-review-draft-report.pdfpetition Commission of Singapore (CCS) (2010) Statement of Decision pursuant to Regulation 9 of the Competition Regulations 2007. Application for Decision by the Singapore Medical Association in relation to its Guideline on Fees pursuant to section 44 of the Competition Act, 18th August http://www.ccs.gov.sg/content/dam/ccs/PDFs/Public_register_and_consultation/Public_register/Anticompetitive_Agreements/SMA-SD%20%2818%20Aug%202010%29.pdf.

Chapter 7

Rational Federalism for Sustainable Public Hospitals[*]

David Gadiel & Jeremy Sammut

The 'blame game' redux

Under Australia's complex federal system, public hospital services are owned and operated by state and territory governments, but are funded jointly. These mixed financial and operational responsibilities mean that a constant feature of the health policy landscape is the 'blame game'. The states blame service delivery problems, including lengthy wait times for emergency and elective public hospital care, on inadequate federal health funding. In response, the federal government attributes these problems to inefficient and ineffective state government public hospital management.

Before the 2007 federal election, then-Opposition leader Kevin Rudd promised to implement national health reforms that would "end the blame game" over public hospitals. Under the new federal health funding agreement eventually negotiated by Prime Minister Julia Gillard in 2011, the federal government agreed to increase its funding for state health services, and the states agreed to a national system of 'activity-based', casemix funding for public hospital services. This means, where possible, that public hospitals are paid for each occasion of service they actually deliver, defined according to casemix (based on separations grouped according to ICD-10-AM into Australian Refined Diagnosis Related Groups), for

* First published as Medi-Mess: Rational Federalism and Patient Cost-Sharing for Public Hospital Sustainability in Australia, Research Report 30, (Sydney: The Centre for Independent Studies, 2017).

which they are remunerated at a 'national efficient price' (based on cost weights allocated in accordance with average variable inputs such as clinical labour, length of stay, etc). Some separations, such as for mental health, are still subject to block grant funding. The so-called 'efficient' price is periodically determined by an Independent Hospital Pricing Authority (IHPA) based on national averages across the public hospital system.[1]

The Gillard government's 'National Partnership' funding formula committed the federal government to fund set proportions of the cost of public hospital care at 44% of the 'efficient' cost of each inpatient public hospital separation by 2020–21. This included 50% of the 'efficient' cost of growth in activity from 2017–18. The agreement meant the federal government was expected to increase hospital funding to the states by $26 billion over the ten years between 2013–14 and 2024–25 — causing its contribution to public hospital funding to rise by 185% from $14 billion to $40 billion.

However, the blame game re-emerged with a vengeance following the change of government from Labor to the Coalition in September 2013. The Abbott government rightly deemed the promise of 50% federal government 'growth funding' to be unaffordable on even the most optimistic projections of future revenue, and especially in the context of seeking to repair the federal budget and reduce the deficit and debt. The Gillard deal and activity-based funding formula was replaced with the standard funding arrangement — a capped, or fixed, annual federal contribution to the cost of state health services, indexed by CPI and for population growth, unrelated to activity.[2] In response to further protests by the states and territories, these decisions have effectively been reversed, in the short-term at least, by the new activity-based growth funding agreement introduced by the Turnbull government covering the period 2017–2020 (see below).[3]

While the Abbott government's 2014 Budget funding changes were presented in the media as an annual 'cut' to hospital funding totalling $50 billion over the 10 years to 2024–25, federal funding for hospitals remained destined to increase to $25 billion by 2024–25. The Coalition had also suggested—via its 2014 *Commission of Audit* and 2015 *Competition Policy Review* processes—that to limit the call on public resources, market-based policies were needed. These included greater involvement of more efficient private sector providers in the delivery of health and hospital services.[4]

The focus on efficiency was understandable. In all jurisdictions, health consumes around a third of the state budget, and public hospitals account for around two-thirds of total health spending. Between 2003–04 and 2013–14, total federal, state and territory government expenditure on public hospitals increased by 80% in real terms, and more than doubled in all states and territories except NSW and Victoria (Figure 8). All states and territories have recorded substantial increases in real spending, and the rising cost of public hospital care has been a major source of pressure on government budgets.[5]

Figure 8: Increase in real recurrent federal, state and territory government expenditure on public hospitals ($ billion)

	2003-04	2013-14	Real increase % *
NSW	$7.78	$13.27	70.5%
Vic	$6.32	$9.75	54.4%
Qld	$3.81	$7.96	108.8%
WA	$2.21	$4.47	102.5%
SA	$1.77	$3.59	102.9%
Tas	$0.44	$0.90	103.6%
ACT	$0.43	$0.96	124.7%
NT	$0.31	$0.73	132.3%
Aust	$23.07	$41.63	80.4%

Sources: Productivity Commission, Report on Government Services 2013, Table 10A.2 & Productivity Commission, Report on Government Services 2016, Table 11A.2

Lack of productivity was a major issue because additional 'inputs' were being absorbed without a proportional increase in 'outputs'† (as is typical in the public sector). This was tacitly acknowledged by the Gillard funding agreement. The creation of a national funding system based on defined hospital 'products', priced on national 'efficiency' criteria, may be used to justify improving public hospital productivity by encouraging them to realise gains at least to reach average levels of efficiency — thereby lowering the overall cost of hospital services to both federal and state budgets.

Dilemma of a 'free' system

The 2011 introduction of the national activity-based funding system appears, at face value, to have had an impact on public hospital finances. But it is hard to distinguish evidence of the impact from the effect of parallel administrative measures to ration access to free care.

As a component of its estimates of Australian health expenditure, the Australian Institute of Health and Welfare (AIHW) shows that over the period 2009-10 to 2014-15, recurrent growth in real public hospital expenditure was 3.4%, compared with 4.4% over the longer period 2004-05 to 2014-15. This compares with a higher comparable growth over the period 2004-05 to 2009-10 of 5.4%, immediately prior to the introduction of activity-based funding.[6] These estimates of comparative expenditure growth are roughly consistent with a heavily qualified, equivalent time series on levels of expenditure in the AIHW's *Hospital Resources* report. However, there is lack of consistent continuous time series data on total recurrent hospital expenditures for the years 2010-11 to 2014-15. Due to the lack of year-to-year consistency in the collection of the latter, the AIHW has declined in this instance to use them to publish figures for the behaviour of expenditure growth—choosing not to calculate figures for average change in recurrent expenditure 'since 2010-11' and 'since 2013-14.'[7]

---

† This problem was well demonstrated by the findings of the 2013 Queensland Commission of Audit headed by Peter Costello. The Commission found that while expenditure on public hospitals in Queensland had 'increased 43% in the five years since 2007, activity increased by less than half — only 17%. Queensland Commission of Audit, Final Report (Brisbane: Government of Queensland, 2013), 22.

Even if we were to admit expenditure data (of better quality than available) as evidence of the impact of activity funding in controlling hospital expenditure growth, we would need to allow for the confounding effect of rationing through use of public hospital waiting lists.

Between 2011-12 and 2014-15, admissions from public hospital elective surgery waiting lists increased by 1.9%; but between 2013-14 and 2014-15 they fell by 0.2%. These figures are more significant given that three-quarters of public hospital surgery is performed in larger public hospitals. Between 2011-12 and 2014-15, admissions from 'principal referral and women's and children's hospitals' and 'public acute group A hospitals' increased by 1.6% and 2.8% respectively; but between 2013-14 and 2014-15 their respective growth rates fell to 0.8% and to 0.6%.[8]

The reduced growth in admissions (which does not take into account increased demand due to population growth and ageing) may indicate activity-based funding has contributed to hospital activity, but to the extent of eventually precipitating a curb on the rate of elective admissions to enable hospitals to remain within overall budget caps. Administrative controls at hospital level (in lieu of price signals) —including patient waits, rationing of surgical lists and temporarily closing operating theatres and wards — can limit access to care and control expenditure (regardless of how hospitals are remunerated) much in the same way as expenditure caps imposed at state or national levels, but they are not a mark of efficiency.

As things stand, the states are still demanding the federal government fully restores the $50 billion 2014 Budget cuts — which would see public hospital expenditure grow well above forecast GDP — or increase the GST rate to 15% to fill the 'funding gap'.[9]

There is no clarity about the impact of activity-based funding on hospital expenditure since 2011. Moreover, there is the likelihood its effect could ultimately prove equivocal in controlling health costs. To the extent it makes resources more productive, activity-based funding (without the distortion of administrative rationing) creates an incentive to treat more patients and increase community access to care. Activity funding may thereby yield health consumption gains that know no bounds—as might be expected of any uncapped fee-for-service payment mechanism.[10] The associated higher service volumes—even if they are remunerated at supposedly efficient prices—could thus cause the total cost of public hospital care to increase. Perversely, but understandably, more efficient and productive public hospitals with more patient throughput will not necessarily prove less expensive. As we shall show, under Medicare funding arrangements (all other things remaining equal) it may in fact cause overall public hospital expenditure to increase.

Box 11 Australian health federalism: 1975, 1984, and thereafter

- State and territory governments have always been responsible for their public health services. But before the 1970s, the federal government had limited involvement in state health and hospital systems. The successful referendum on social services in 1946 gave the federal government the authority to fund state-run health services. Under the National Health Scheme of the Menzies government of the 1950s, federal government 'hospital benefits' were made available to the states to contribute to the cost of public hospital care. Prior to this in 1942, the states had agreed to refer their constitutional power to levy income taxes to the federal government, which levied the first uniform national income tax in return for offering the states what appeared to be a financially attractive funding deal — a portent of the health policy upheavals of the 1970s and thereafter.[11]

- In the 1950s, membership of a private health fund was mandatory to be eligible to receive federal government hospital benefits — a policy that led to around 85% of Australians either being covered by private insurance, or having their health care paid for by the federal government-funded Pensioner Medical Service. A safety net for the disadvantaged unable to afford private health premiums took the form of free, means-tested public hospital care. The federal government benefit was paid to patients as a rebate through their health funds, not to state governments. In combination with fund benefits, this covered the cost of treatment in public hospitals, and offset the (still considerable) operational grants that state governments provided.[12] In essence, however, public hospital services actually rendered were remunerated by a dual private and public financed 'activity' payment system, ensuring a guaranteed 'steady and reliable' flow of clinically-based income and minimal waits for treatment.[13]

- But this was no golden age of public hospitals. State governments continued to struggle with the interrelated problems of funding and

202

governing their hospital services: each public hospital was independently administrated by their own board of governors, but with the state holding ultimate financial responsibility for budget overruns. Public hospitals were a major public administration challenge, since hospital boards frequently overran their budgets and left the state to underwrite the bill. The challenges of achieving financial control and containing the cost of health to state budgets set the stage for the introduction of Medibank (forerunner to Medicare) by the Whitlam Labor government in the mid-1970s.

- In 1975, the federal government offered to share the recurrent net operating costs of public hospitals with state governments on a 50/50, open-ended, dollar-for-dollar basis. This is to say, the Whitlam government persuaded the states to sign up to Medibank — and to agree to provide 'free' public hospital care — by committing the federal government to pay for 50% of real cost of providing all the public hospital services demanded and delivered each year, without rationing, queues, and waiting lists. The promise of having their mouths stuffed with gold and alleviating the financial burdens imposed by public hospitals was an offer the states could not refuse — and turned out to be too good to be true.[14]

- The Whitlam promise quickly proved unaffordable. The cost-sharing arrangement was immediately scrapped by the Coalition government under Prime Minister Malcolm Fraser, which agreed instead to fund only 50% of hospital costs 'approved' in consultation in the states. In 1981, the federal government withdrew entirely from the cost-sharing arrangement, which was replaced with 'identified' (fixed or capped) health grants to the states, and was justified on the grounds of making the states more financially accountable. When the Hawke government re-branded and re-introduced Medibank as Medicare in 1984, it extended the Fraser government's approach and continued to limit the federal government financial exposure to the cost of 'free' public hospital care by giving the states only capped health grants.

- Given the intractable vertical fiscal imbalance in the federation - the division of health policy and funding responsibilities was far from ideal. The federal government, with the bulk of the taxing powers, was not responsible for financing anything like the actual cost of the real demand for public hospital care. The Whitlam promise of Canberra paying 50% of the real operating cost of 'free' public hospital care was the fool's gold. Though no federal government under Hawke, Keating, Howard, Rudd, Gillard, Abbott, or Turnbull was ever close to fulfilling this promise — the federal share of hospital costs has traditionally hovered somewhere around 40% of the total cost of (rationed) public hospital services — the states have been committed to delivering 'free' hospital care with major budgetary and political consequences.[15]

The imperfect path to public hospital expenditure control since 1984

Since the establishment of Medicare in 1984, the federal government has funded state and territory health services on the condition that public hospital care is delivered to all Australians without charge at the point of consumption. This rigid and onerous obligation to guarantee universal free access has exposed states to the risk of paying for unlimited free public hospital care. Without price signals, there is a presumption that demand will inevitably grow faster than supply. The ability to access free hospital services creates moral hazard. There is a risk of over-use and over-servicing, with unlimited demand for separations matching (if not overwhelming) any efficiency gains. Because increases in supply can never be fully accommodated, the efficiency gain may be lost to inflated and wasteful health expenditure.

The states' financial exposure to the cost of public hospitals has been heightened because federal health funding has always been capped (never demand-driven) to limit the federal government's financial obligations. Federal government funding for state health services has also been capped to offset the increasing cost of its open-ended, on-demand, 'own program' Medicare fee-for-service expenditure on the Medical Benefits Scheme (MBS) and Pharmaceutical Benefits Scheme (PBS).[16] Federal government funding for state health services has thus dwindled in real terms since Medicare's inception.[17] Moreover, the federal government has the majority of taxing powers in the federation. This includes full power over income tax. During World War II the states relinquished—but did not abandon—their constitutional power to levy income tax to the federal government. The resulting chronic vertical fiscal imbalance in the Australian federation - the disparity between the federal government's control over the majority of taxing powers (including power over income tax), and fiscal demands placed upon states and territories to assume health and other service responsibilities - means the states' ability to meet their responsibilities has remained heavily dependent on the federal government; and since 2000, on the share of the federal government-levied Goods and Services Tax (GST) revenue distributed to each state and territory.

The federation's disparity between revenue powers and health service responsibilities, combined with the federal government's overarching control of the health policy framework, means the states have legitimate grievances about federal-state financial relations in executing their public hospital services management and delivery responsibilities. But the story in health is more complicated than the simplistic blame game over 'lack of money'.

In the mid-1970s, state governments were promised that creation of a universal, taxpayer-funded national health scheme would alleviate the funding and governance burdens associated with operating public hospitals, because the federal government would bear half the real cost of 'free' hospital care—a promise never fulfilled (Box 11). In reality, the coming of Medicare has left the states in financial straits.

State governments with relatively small and independent sources of revenue, and large and competing service delivery obligations, have shouldered the financial consequences of increasing public hospital use. This began when a large fall in private health fund membership was precipitated by the establishment of Medicare and the end of the public hospital means test. This shifted the full cost of treatment for formerly privately-insured patients onto state government budgets. PHI coverage fell from 64% of the population in 1983, to 47% in the late 1980s, to 30% in the late 1990s. The rate recovered to 47% only following the introduction of 'Lifetime Cover' rules, the PHI tax rebate, and Medicare surcharge arrangements by the Howard government in the early 2000s.

Since 1984, financial realities have forced state governments to make hard decisions about access to 'free' public hospital care. The predictable response—to limit the threat of Medicare unleashing unlimited health expenditure on over-stretched state budgets—was to implement blunt expenditure controls. These consisted of frontline 'global' budget caps that bore little relationship to the actual demand for 'free' care, but which rationed access to services (chiefly by cutting hospital bed numbers and surgical lists). This in turn, led to the emergence and blowouts in waiting times for emergency and elective treatment.[18]

Given that states have severely limited macro-political authority over health, they sought to control their share of the cost of Medicare by rationing services. Rationing by queuing was achieved by funding hospitals through the traditional block payment mechanism, with funding caps imposed to restrict operational capacity and limit the amount of care provided. Rationing was implemented in conjunction with governance changes that centralised financial and operational control over hospitals in state health departments — an administrative structure that has compromised the efficiency of public hospital systems (see below).

To minimise waiting times and enhance financial control over public hospitals, activity-based funding was introduced initially in Victoria in 1993,[19] and thereafter indicatively, or in piecemeal fashion, in other jurisdictions. Supply-side initiatives — in general, and including effectively designed activity based funding (if strictly enforced) — can be important to address productivity lags and enhance policymakers' ability to achieve the best value for taxpayers' dollars by extracting the maximum level of services obtainable from available health resources. State government-led microeconomic reform initiatives to the extent the Medicare framework permits, including outsourcing delivery of publicly-funded hospital care to private operators where possible, can also partly mitigate governance (or public sector management) issues that impede public hospital performance.

In this vein, the national activity-based funding system may be interpreted as an exercise in seeking 'efficient' terms on which the proportion of hospital costs are distributed between federal and state budgets. It is likely to have an impact on the unit-cost of care and on waiting times by using resources more intensively and productively — but most likely restricted to the least efficient hospitals (Box 12). A more justifiable supply-side option would simply have been to define unit outputs according to casemix criteria and to permit hospitals to compete on price within an 'internal market'. The very notion of a 'national efficient price' conveys something of a Stakhanovite flavour.

In any event, the new funding system will not alter the fundamentals of a 'free' system, or eliminate blame shifting over waits and funding. The blame game will continue while ever the federal government continues to write blank cheques for 'free' hospital care that the states can never hope to cash. While the existing Medicare framework remains, rationing of access to hospital care by queuing will remain an unavoidable feature of a 'free' system, with total budget and service limits imposed by state health department 'system managers' to contain the cost to the public purse.

The real problem with Australia's public hospitals is that federal involvement in state health systems has jeopardised state finances. However efficiently hospital services are produced, it is simply unaffordable for governments to pay for 'free' hospital care on demand. Certainly, activity-based funding may help accommodate an increasing demand for public hospital services caused by an ageing and growing population and new medical technology,[20] because there is a presumption that higher volumes of services can be delivered for a given quantity of health funding. But paying public hospitals at what purports to be the efficient price does not guarantee their financial sustainability in an ageing Australia, since states must fund larger outputs of hospital services at zero prices. When hospitals exceed their budgets, there is always a risk of states having to bail them out by supplementing their share of activity funding from other state budgetary sources (Box 12). When this occurs, it saps the incentive for managers to improve efficiency and defeats the purpose of activity funding. There will hence always be the risk of efficiency gains being squandered on unnecessary or excessive services in feeding (at zero prices) an infinitely elastic demand for hospital care that is underwritten by ballooning state expenditure.

Box 12. Centrally-planned technical inefficiency

- Enforcing budget caps and rationing care, as necessitated by Medicare, required altering the governance arrangements of public hospitals by centralising financial and administrative control over hospitals in state health departments. Local hospital boards were abolished and 'area health' authorities were established to administer hospitals in designated regions. This command-and-control structure involves detailed micro-

---

management of day-to-day hospital activities and centralised setting of policies (especially of industrial agreements) by remote centralised agencies. This has made public hospital systems by-words for bureaucracy and high administrative overheads, and resulted in well-documented negative effects on hospital management, efficiency and costs — lengthening waiting times by compromising the ability of the public system to deliver timely and cost-effective care.[21]

- The need for devolution of independent and accountable management responsibility to the local level has been a policy goal articulated for many years by state and federal politicians. Regrettably, in practice this has not been achieved, despite periodic and repeated redesign of governance arrangements. Instead, public hospitals in all jurisdictions continue to be run as branch offices of state health departments, which operate as both the funder and provider of centrally coordinated hospital services. Though public hospitals are currently under the nominal control of 'Local Health District' (LHD) agencies and their government-appointed boards of directors, state health departments remain the 'system managers' and retain high levels of involvement in the operational affairs of hospitals.[22]

- The principal reason for continuing with highly centralised hospital management is because state treasuries carry the financial risk for the operating budgets of public hospitals. These governance arrangements — despite being subject to perennial and persistent criticism — have proved impervious to change. This is because, ultimately, the financial risk for 'free' hospital care is carried by the purchaser (state governments) not the provider — individual hospitals, which remain responsible to health departments whose primary task is to try to prevent or limit budget overruns.

- In practice, this environment creates a public sector monopoly that guarantees public hospitals will receive government custom, while dulling incentives for operational efficiency and good management, since public hospitals are not properly accountable for their financial performance. Because standard practice is for additional allocations to be made by Treasury to cover operating deficits, there is no real requirement for hospital managers to exert proper control over hospital finances. This can make a mockery of 'national efficient pricing', which is the hallmark of activity funding, because it is always open to states to effectively underwrite higher prices by increasing their share of the funding. In addition to undermining financial accountability, centralisation also impedes productivity and innovation, due to the lack of independent management. Frontline managers are expected to meet centrally mandated KPIs, but have limited managerial autonomy and prerogatives, and little ability to overcome workplace rigidities that impede the efficient operation of public hospitals.

- Centralised control of human resources has invited provider 'capture' in the form of high labour cost, inefficient work practices and rigid demarcations that impede cost-effective management and efficient delivery of quality hospital care. Many restrictive work practices are entrenched by state-wide industrial agreements between health departments and powerful health trade unions (including ASMOF, controlled by the Australian Medical Association, and the Australian Nursing Federation) which set the terms and conditions for employment for doctors, nurses, and allied health professionals. Hospital managers seeking innovative ways to deliver hospital care lack authority over their clinical workforces; multi-skilling, task-substitution and redeployment of the clinical workforce are prohibited by rigid demarcations inherent in industrial agreements.

- State-wide nursing awards, combined with the freedoms visiting medical officers (VMOs) and staff specialists may exercise over their own schedules and work practices, deny managers the flexibility to secure efficient and effective care. Nursing is the largest single area of recurrent hospital cost, and nurses' awards uniformly fix scales of remuneration across the entire state as well as conditions of employment that protect public nursing jobs — such as the strict nurse-to-patient ratios of one nurse per four patients that are a standard feature of nurse award conditions across Australia and a major barrier to productivity. Nurse-to-patient ratios exacerbate staff shortages, raise costs, and limit patient throughput because inefficiently using a hospital's nursing workforce limits the number of beds available.

- Hence the so-called 'national efficient price' terminology associated with the national activity-based funding system is a misnomer. The so-called efficient price is calculated by averaging the cost across all services, which means the national activity-based funding system will implicitly under-write the existing inefficiencies embedded in the public hospital system. It would help to discover the true efficient price of public hospital services and deliver the best value for the ever-increasing amount of taxpayers' money spent if the kind of structural reforms that have been commonplace in other government instrumentalities in the last 30 years were implemented. However, state governments have been reluctant to undertake them in relation to public hospitals for fear of the political repercussions.

Medicare is the problem

According to the 2016 NSW Government Inter-Generational Report, the rising cost of 'efficient' public hospital services is unsustainable. The report shows that under current tax and health policy settings, by 2055–56 rising health expenditure—driven mainly by the increasing cost of public hospital care to the NSW budget—will be responsible for 60% of the forecast 'fiscal gap' between revenue and expenditure of 3.4% of Gross State Product.[23] Former NSW premier Mike Baird described health funding as an "unbelievable challenge and the numbers continue to be daunting."[24] In response, the NSW Government has led calls by state governments for the federal parliament to increase the rate of GST from 10% to 15% to fund (in part at least) the state health burden.[25] This would represent the largest peacetime increase in taxation in Australian history and is an indication of the scale of the 'hospital funding crisis'.

The federal government's Inter-Generational Report (IGR) also shows the rising cost of health in coming decades will be primarily responsible for placing unbearable fiscal pressure on the federal budget—necessitating either substantial tax rises, cuts to services, larger deficits and debts, or their combination.[26] Ironically, the fiscal projections in the IGR exclude the impact of current federal policy on state budgets—even though the federal government, as architect of Medicare, is imperilling state and territory public hospital systems.

For more than three decades, state and territory governments of all persuasions have struggled to operate 'free' public hospitals effectively amid rising demand, escalating community expectations, and growing public dissatisfaction. In the long run, public hospital services are unaffordable under current policy settings. No level of government, state or federal, with or without activity funding, will have sufficient money to pay for the projected cost of all the 'free' hospital care the community will want to consume out of taxes it is willing and able to pay. Therefore, what is fundamentally unsustainable about the Australian public hospital system is the federally-mandated policy of 'free' public hospital care that has prevailed since the start of Medicare in 1984. The operation of Medicare has prevented state governments from taking effective remedial action to address jointly the supply-side defects with the demand-side issues critical to the sustainability of hospital services.

Because 'free' health care has become a 'sacred cow', too little attention has been paid to the role Medicare has played in creating the public hospital 'mess'. The irreconcilable policy objectives of increasing 'free' access, while containing the cost of a 'free' system, is a dilemma that state governments understandably find impossible to solve under the existing health policy settings.

The standard view in health public policy circles is that a uniform national health policy is intrinsically meritorious. The principle of subsidiarity — that full policy, funding, and political responsibility should reside with the level of government closest to the point of service — is consequently sacrificed to the populist cause of 'free' public hospital treatment.

Another view is that federal government meddling in state public hospital systems since 1984 has created the public hospital mess by imposing on state governments the Sisyphean task of delivering 'free' hospital care to all comers, while restricting the states' policy authority over their hospitals. This has created unintended but predictable consequences, including rationing and related governance and productivity issues that have compromised the performance of state hospital systems. The need to contain the financial risk inherent in a 'free' system has contributed to high levels of bureaucracy with centralised state health department control over the daily activities of public hospitals. This has bequeathed a command-and-control structure that — in combination with productivity-killing, state-wide industrial agreements covering a highly unionised clinical workforce — thwarts independent, accountable and innovative management at the local level. (Box 12)

Even if states summoned the political will to undertake meaningful microeconomic reform to address governance problems, improving the productivity and technical efficiency of public hospitals (Box 13), this would be insufficient to ensure the long-term future of public hospitals and the solvency of state budgets. The affordability challenges in state health systems cannot reduce simply to states applying sound principles of public administration. There are underlying structural causes that have been exacerbated over the last three decades by federal interference in state hospital systems, associated with the service responsibilities of Medicare. The blame game over the inadequacies of federal funding for health has gifted states a perpetual excuse to not confront overdue microeconomic reform.[27] Yet this should not distract from the role that federal-state financial relations inherent in Medicare have played in creating the public hospital mess.

A comprehensive solution to the public hospital crisis requires a federalist solution that will resolve the public hospital mess by permitting states to address not only the supply-side challenges in a meaningful way, but also to deal with the crucial demand-side challenges. This requires new federal-state financial relations that will safeguard state budgets by allowing states to assume simultaneous control over public hospital funding, policy and service responsibilities.

Federalism and demand-side reform

Revision of the federation to end federal meddling in state health systems through national control of health policy could play a constructive role in encouraging states to make rational decisions about health policy. The key to creating affordable public hospital systems is to endow the states with sufficient authority and incentive to make these decisions—and to take their electorates with them towards sustainable health and hospital systems. As we have remarked above, this requires realignment at the state level between financial (tax) policy and political and health service responsibilities. States and territories have yet to comprehend it is in their best interest for the federal authorities to cease dictating health policy and to take back their income tax responsibilities, recognising, as this report argues, that taxing and service responsibilities should go hand in hand.

The states' reluctance to seek or accept a return of these responsibilities was evidenced when Prime Minister Malcolm Turnbull sought in vain to germinate his model of 'competitive federalism', announced as a curtain raiser to the COAG meeting with state leaders in April 2016.

The Prime Minister proposed that the federal government would reduce the federal income tax by an agreed percentage to allow the states to levy an income tax equal to that amount, thereby enabling the termination of existing federal grant programs such as funding for state hospital services. This 'tax swap' idea was based on a proposal canvassed in 2014 by the Abbott government's National Commission of Audit, which suggested that the marginal rate of federal income tax be cut from 32.5% to 22.5% to allow the states to collect the remaining 10% as a "state income tax surcharge".[28] As the then Prime Minister rightly argued, a state income tax would address the central conflict: the inability of a state directly to raise revenue sufficient for their own responsibilities, while making them directly accountable to voters and taxpayers in their states for how revenue was spent. While there would initially be no overall increase in taxation, in the longer term a state income tax would also enable states to exercise financial autonomy with freedom to increase or lower taxation as necessary—ending once and for all the blame game over federal-state financial relations.[29]

When the states rejected the tax swap deal, the hospital funding can was kicked down the road for political reasons. To remove the issue from the agenda ahead of the 2016 federal election, the Turnbull government struck an interim Heads of Agreement with the states that restored some of the 'savings' cut from the Gillard funding deal by the 2014 budget. For a period of three years from 1 July 2017 to 30 June 2020, the federal government agreed to fund 45% of the efficient growth of activity-based services, with overall growth in federal funding capped at 6.5% (in line with the reduction of growth in hospital costs under the national activity-based funding system), with a longer-term funding deal to be negotiated and to commence thereafter.[30] The deal was subsequently supplemented by an additional commitment by the Turnbull Government of $2.8 billion over the four-year forward estimates announced in the 2017 Budget. [31]

The outcome of the April 2016 COAG meeting—along with the Turnbull government's subsequent abandonment of the White Paper on Reform of the Federation—suggests recasting federalism is unlikely to proceed through a top-down, Procrustean approach imposed from above. Instead, such initiatives may perhaps ultimately more plausibly be instigated from below—that is, by the states facing reality about the unsustainability of the federal-state health and financial relations status quo.

The rejection of federalism is a paradox: it shows state governments have yet to understand how their best interests would have been served by levying a state income tax to fund their health services.

To avoid the financial calamity of fundamentally unsustainable free hospital systems that no government—state or federal—can afford, states should therefore honestly confront the unsustainability of the federal-state health and financial relations status quo. Reform of the federation can be driven only from the bottom up. State governments must lead the way on reform of the federation to safeguard their own budgets from Medicare, and to endow themselves with the means to undertake the demand-side policies key to sustainable hospital services.

States should therefore demand the right and opportunity to take back their income tax powers—equivalent initially to the quantum of hospital funding they would sacrifice as specific purpose grants and the federal government share of activity funding, met from federal government tax collections. The percentage of the federal income tax scales so surrendered would thereafter be designated 'state income tax', including the Medicate levy.

The method of its collection would remain the same, with both the state and federal income tax collected by the Australian Taxation Office (ATO). However, the extent of income tax raised on behalf of participating states could rise or fall as necessary to meet their health and other service responsibilities. The political responsibility for the state income tax rate would encourage reform in health on the supply-side (as above), as well as focus attention on the demand-side policy dilemma still confronting public hospitals.

The logical corollary of a state's decision to reclaim its income tax powers would effectively release it from its obligation under Medicare to provide free public hospital care. But after the debacle of April 2016, to advocate for such reform may even charitably be interpreted as 'courageous'. Tampering with the fundamentals of Medicare is the third rail of Australian politics. Yet the feasibility and case for restoring state income tax, in conjunction with public hospital charging, needs to be assessed in light of its unpalatable alternatives.

Even if states were to embark upon microeconomic reform, supply-side initiatives and productivity gains can never in themselves suffice to sustain public hospital Medicare. We have shown how the effect of unconstrained demand in a more supply-side efficient, but 'free', hospital system would be more expensive. It would perpetuate—and possibly intensify—the need to contain costs by rationing with queuing or bailing out inferior hospital management. Further, supply-side reform as a stand-alone policy without price signals would inevitably create a vortex for further spiralling demand excesses, augmented by the impact of population ageing and advances in medical technology.

The sustainability of public hospitals can be addressed ultimately only with demand-side initiatives as an ingredient in reform and as a component of rational federalism—which Medicare now precludes. State governments accordingly need to address this by reasserting their income tax powers in conjunction with a release from the requirement to deliver 'free' public hospital care. Restoration of full financial and policy responsibility for public hospitals would allow states discretion in designing their own strategies for their own hospitals' public policy, subject as always to the will of the electorate.

Rational federalism would invite state governments to seek political support for local income taxes to fund public hospitals. There is a presumption that state leaders would already have been in 'hard' conversation with their electorates about the future of their public hospital systems. Once adopted, state income tax would become an immediate spur to hospital efficiency.

Fear of increasing state income tax to cover the cost of badly managed hospitals would encourage local politicians not only to make effective decisions about how to run public hospitals, but also to adopt realistic dialogue with voters about the real demand-side challenges.

Many states already make it their business to charge for public hospital care, but as revenue measures, wherever the letter of the law permits.[33] At admission, all patients are routinely exhorted to elect to be treated as private, fee-paying patients (even in emergency situations), especially where it can be established that they possess an entitlement to third-party payer support such as private health insurance, workers' compensation or a motor accident or tort liability claim. Most patients who incur fees thus willingly accept a double cost burden. As taxpayers under Medicare, everyone pays for their free hospital entitlement but any private fees additionally incurred represent a further layer of direct or indirect charges, depending upon any right of recourse to claim a private benefit.

Miscellaneous charges, such as to Medicare-ineligible patients and for outpatient pharmaceutical charges, are meticulously enforced; hospital car parking operates at full capacity on commercial principles and attracts high charges from franchise operators that customers are evidently willing to pay as a proxy co-payment (although starting in July 2017, the NSW government is proposing to introduce concessions for certain patients and carers); ambulance fees apply to the general population and may be pursued through debt collection agencies if necessary. Charging by public hospitals is thus extensively employed; it represents a boundary already crossed. The pathway to wider adoption of this principle may not be as far-reaching as its critics will try to claim.

If more formally, widely and explicitly adopted, charging for all public hospital care as a demand-side policy, rather than as a purely revenue measure, would become self-reinforcing. States would clearly be reluctant to turn back the clock to wear the political odium of perpetually drip-feeding unconstrained hospital utilisation (of doubtful health gain) with higher state income taxes or debt or both. Rather, they would be encouraged to continue to court electoral favour with lower taxation. This would reinforce effective hospital policy embodying supply side and managerial efficiency with minimal patient waiting times. The extent of hospital charges that patients cost-shared would reflect the efficiencies realised. States would be better placed to retire their debt, lower their income taxes and thereby to provide a magnet for population increase, private investment and economic growth.

Not all jurisdictions may have an appetite for the discipline of a state income tax—let alone demand-side hospital reform. A more palatable alternative could be an 'opt-out' approach that might permit states individually and voluntarily to assert their income tax powers and to reclaim authority over health policy to pursue their own path in budgetary and hospital system sustainability (Box 14).

The benefits of economic growth in states that adopted these new fiscal principles would deliver them greater capacity (through all tax collected) to support the delivery of high quality health services and to open new opportunities for innovative hospitals operating in generally more contestable settings.

On the other hand, states not introducing their own income tax and who neglected the chance to embark on rational hospital management strategies would be confronted with the risk of ensuing 'backwash' effects of economic growth in states participating in reform. States opting for the status quo would ultimately feel obliged to consider competing with reformist jurisdictions by synchronising for themselves the adoption of state income taxes linked to hospital policy reform. Alternatively, they could risk their investment and economic growth stagnating. The re-birthing of health financing could, moreover, provide a blueprint for financial reform in other high-spending portfolios for which states are responsible, such as education, that—like hospitals—have become addicted to federal funding as a matter of expedience.

Box 13. Microeconomic reform

- The supply-side strategies that can address the interrelated governance and productivity problems in public hospitals are well-known. These entail a three-stage microeconomic reform agenda involving: (1) Creating a purchaser-provider split; (2) Corporatising public hospitals with truly independent and accountable boards; (3) Introducing competition and contestability (competitive pricing) via privatisation or corporatisation of public hospital facilities[32].

- Reorientating the system towards market-based arrangements requires transforming the traditional role of state health departments into purchasers of hospital services. Instead of acting as both funder and provider of centrally coordinated hospital services as under the existing public monopoly model, central agencies should instead act as informed and discriminating purchasers, responsible for negotiating service agreements and contracts with local hospitals, with the ability to direct custom (without sacrifice to quality care) to better performing hospitals to contain expenditure and maximise the state's return on health spending.

- The first stage of microeconomic reform — a legitimate, arms-length purchaser-provider split arrangement — depends on the second stage: the meaningful devolution of financial and managerial authority via privatisation or corporatisation of public hospitals. This requires devolving managerial and financial responsibility (including financial risk) for each public hospital to their own board of management, with full control over all operational matters and full responsibility for the hospital's entire budget. Incentives for operational efficiency would be enhanced if budgetary responsibility, including financial risk for 'core' clinical services (covering nurses, doctors and allied health), were carried (at least in part) by the provider instead of the purchaser (the state government). This could be achieved by emulating the ideals of the Foundation Trust hospital governance model of the National Health Service in England. Foundation Trust boards have the power to borrow and are responsible for debt incurred and can accumulate reserves as a reward for efficiency. Their solvency is monitored by an independent regulator. Trusts nevertheless have been marred by chronic insufficient capacity to meet burgeoning demand at NHS zero prices. (Independent administrators, for example, were obliged to take over the Mid Staffs Foundation Trust in 2013 to avert its insolvency).

- Ideally, each hospital board and CEO would have full administrative and budgetary control and be responsible for setting the price of its services in competition with other private and public facilities. Importantly, managerial autonomy and financial accountability under a corporatised system of hospital governance would mean giving hospital managers full control over the employment terms and conditions of their workforces. Independent managerial authority would include the freedom to negotiate enterprise agreements with staff that take local conditions and financial realities into account. Workplace flexibility would eliminate restrictive and inappropriate 'one size fits all' industrial agreements, and facilitate the implementation of innovative ways of delivering cost-effective services—a process encouraged by the incentives created by financial accountability and competition.

- A purchaser-provider split would also allow for a new model of private sector involvement in the delivery of public hospital services. Selective privatisation via Public Private Partnerships, for new or redevelopment hospital projects, would create a competitive and contestable market for public hospital services, and give state health departments the ability to act with discretion as informed purchasers of all capital and variable inputs, including clinical labour. The ability to purchase services from better performing operators in contestable environments would encourage public facilities that remained in state hands to lift their performance and to emulate the more efficient and business-like practices of privatised or corporatised competitors. Microeconomic reform has the potential to deliver greater efficiency gains by encouraging the adoption of business axioms usually foreign to public hospitals. These include a culture of competition and innovation; more efficient, customer-focused service delivery; more flexible health labour work practices; and superior managerial accountability.

- State governments should no longer allow public hospitals to be quarantined from structural reform. Political will is needed to confront and dilute the vested interests of health labour employed in public hospitals that has long benefited from government-funded public hospital employment on privileged terms. The introduction of market disciplines and incentives into the public hospital sector would improve productivity and encourage innovations that lower costs and improve quality. As in other areas of the economy subject to structural reform, the community would receive more and better hospital services for what — as the cost pressures of coming decades become apparent — will be our increasingly scarce health dollars. A microeconomic reform agenda will therefore help to control escalating health expenditure, improve access and increase the volume of services at least cost.

Box 14: An opt-out model for federalism reform

- Achieving universal agreement among the states on reform of the federation would be difficult. In the absence of consensus, one solution could allow states individually and voluntarily to reclaim their income tax powers and authority over health policy, in conjunction with a tax swap with the federal government. However, this would involve the federal government striking differential rates of income taxes across states. This would be unconstitutional: sections 99 and 51(ii) of the Australian Constitution prohibit unequal treatment of states by the Commonwealth with respect to taxation.

- Optional reform of the federation, state-by-state, in an indirect but constitutionally valid form would still be possible. For states acting alone, this could be done if the federal government were to agree to:

  A. Convert the existing federal specific purpose payment for state health services into a general purpose payment. This would simultaneously release the state from its Medicare obligation to provide free public hospital care inherent in the conditions of the specific purpose grant.

  B. Index the general purpose payment to the amount of health funding the state would otherwise receive according to the formula used to distribute health funding to other states.

  C. Identify the value of the general purpose payment with the equivalent percentage of federal income tax revenue collected in the state. This would become the 'public hospital levy' in all but name.

  D. A state could, if it wished, supplement the federal public hospital levy either by imposing its own income tax surcharge or levy or by issuing a tax rebate under its own legislation but administered by the ATO.

- The opt-out federalism model proposed here has the potential to achieve the following beneficial outcomes:

  1. Establishing an indexed general purpose 'health' grant transparently linked to a specified percentage of the federal income tax collected in the state would end the blame game by making it clear that the citizens of the opt-out state were paying for public hospitals. The percentage of federal income tax so identified as the de facto 'public hospital levy' would represent the real cost of operating public hospitals. Publication of the real public hospital levy would immediately make the state more accountable to voters for how this money was spent on public hospitals.

2. Under an opt-out model, the restoration of state accountability for health would be further enhanced if participating states chose to supplement the federal public hospital levy with their own additional surcharge through a state income tax, as their needs dictated. A hospital surcharge would give opt-out states powerful political incentives to undertake supply- and demand-side reforms. On the other hand, opt-out states would win voter acclaim were they to reduce income tax or perhaps rebate part of federal income tax/state hospital levy to taxpayers as an 'efficiency dividend' for operating sustainable hospital systems. Attention could be drawn to the extent of the gain that each household could derive by specifically inviting them to claim the hospital efficiency rebate as part of their annual tax return.

Strategy for implementing hospital cost sharing

Demand-side health policy in states introducing state income tax could include various forms of patient cost-sharing. However, the default 'roadmap' for these jurisdictions would highlight at least two immediate imperatives.

First, patients exercising their right to public hospital treatment as public patients—including for any form of non-inpatient care that had previously carried an entitlement to admission or treatment without charge under Medicare—would henceforth be obliged to face a compulsory co-payment at the point of consumption. The impact of this would be designed to remove the distortion that (publicly available) insurance introduced between insured hospital services and other health services that may be equally effective. It would cause health service users to adopt greater rationality in their use of hospital services—for example, by perhaps seeking a second opinion for non-emergency elective surgery, or by substituting alternative non-hospital care.

Second, as purely a demand management policy, the intention should be to employ hospital co-payments as far as possible as a 'revenue neutral' measure for both governments and households to pre-empt equity and electoral concerns. This could be achieved by automatically paying quarterly compensation to all households in the state, equivalent to the actuarial cost of a typical household's expected public hospital co-payment disbursements. These payments would reflect the probability of public hospital use, with the amount calibrated according to the characteristics of the household—regardless of whether or not the household had actually accessed any public hospital services (much in the same way as Centrelink at the time of writing paid an analogously-calculated compensatory Energy Supplement to all eligible households in Australia). The cost of the compensation may be amortised with the revenue generated by the co-payment (depending upon the price elasticity of demand for hospital services at prices above zero). And the co-payment's deadweight welfare loss would be minimised to the extent of households substituting other goods for hospital services and other lower-cost care (such as GP or other primary care services) for inpatient care or other hospital services.

Automatic compensation paid to all state residents would minimise the risk of compulsory co-payments for public hospital treatment being branded as unfair, regressive or inequitable. It would preserve the Medicare principle of 'universality' for public hospital treatment since compensation would not be means tested, thereby minimising the risk of political backlash. Compulsory co-payments for hospital services feature in some European national health systems including in France,[34] but they are not compensated (or claimable from health insurance). The French *forfait hospitalier*, for instance, is a daily fee for the "hotel services" component of acute public and private hospital stays. It is currently set at €18 per day (AUD27). This could serve as a model for hospital co-payments in Australia.[35]

Universal hospital co-payments for which everybody is compensated would be politically superior to the Abbott government's ill-fated co-payment plan. Although this exempted low-income groups, it was perceived as violating the principle of 'universality' of entitlement that was originally designed to support the integrity and quality of Medicare. It also encountered a strong electoral backlash from voters resentful of having to contribute directly out of their own pockets to the cost of health services already funded by taxes.[36]

Private treatment in a public hospital would remain charged and paid for as under existing arrangements without attracting a further layer of compensatory entitlement. However, for consistency between publicly and privately insured hospital services, participating states would need to ensure (with federal government approval) first-dollar coverage was banned for all private health insurance tables offered by registered benefit organisations for any form of private care in both public or private hospitals. Health funds would thus need to amend their rules to eliminate gap payments for services related to private patient admissions, including for accommodation, theatre fees, prostheses and specialist medical and laboratory services. All such services would henceforth become subject to specified mandatory co-payments or other acceptable forms of cost sharing. Just as for enhancing the integrity of the public system, the application of like measures to private patients analogously would provide for greater stability in health insurance contribution rates.

Further, for private admissions to public hospitals, abolition of first dollar coverage tables would introduce uniformity and equity between co-payments incurred by public and private patients. For private hospital admissions, co-payments would reduce the risk of patients substituting first-dollar covered private hospital treatment for treatment that would have otherwise occurred privately in a public hospital. In the short run, had it deflected the private caseload away from public hospitals, this may have created more space for treating public patients in public hospitals. However, any such short-lived gain would be likely more than offset by a substantial escalation in health insurance contribution rates—especially in NSW which carries a much larger private patient caseload in public hospitals than other states—since it is much cheaper for health funds to write benefits for private treatment in public hospitals than for equivalent care in private hospitals (to the extent that it is offered in private hospitals).

If higher premiums were precipitated, private insurance coverage may fall, further reinforced in turn by a consequential deterioration of the risk pool of privately insureds, and so on—thereby exposing the public hospital system

223

to the spiralling burden of a growing population disenchanted with health insurance and deflected into public care.

Lessons from Singapore

In summary, for states that were to adopt it, rational federalism could introduce profound changes to their health economies. If properly implemented, it could transcend political resistances and priority would immediately attach to synchronising hospital supply- and demand-side efficiency measures that would permanently change the character of 'hospital Medicare'. Singapore (as Chapter 8 explains) provides an example of a high-income country with extremely good health outcomes. An important part of Singapore's success derives from policies aimed at making patients conscious of the cost of their health services through cost-sharing.

Singapore spends some 4% of its GDP on health, compared with 9% in Australia for the same or better health outcomes. Gadiel and Sammut have shown that Singapore's efficiency is in part attributable to its distinctive health system, the centrepiece of which is a national system of account-based, contributory, personal Health Savings Accounts (HSAs). These are tax-effective savings vehicles that can be used to pay for health services and health insurance,[37] administered through Singapore's Central Provident Fund (CPF).

High levels of personal financial accountability for health expenditure, mandated by use of prices at point of consumption, differentiate Singapore's health system from the likes of Australia's. In Singapore, individuals are required to fund minor health costs for GP care, allied health services, and basic medicines as out-of-pocket expenses. The extensive use of direct patient charges is complemented by the use of insurance deductibles and co-payments for all inpatient care, charged to HSAs, with households thereby sharing in the cost of all hospital services.[38]

The design of Singapore's HSAs has assisted in the extremely effective use of its hospital system through more effective pricing of hospital services at the point of consumption. For example, its hospital separation rate per person year of 0.08 compares favourably with 0.4 in Australia; and the respective comparative hospital bed days used per person year are 0.51 and 2.36.[39] The opportunity for HSAs to play a role in Australian health reform, and for states that adopted 'rational federalism' to offer HSAs as an additional element in hospital cost sharing, is explored in Chapter 8.

Ask not what public hospitals can do for you...

To advocate for HSAs is to emphasise how they can ultimately contribute to household savings. Health reform can thus be presented not simply as confiscating 'free' health care from voters in the name of government budgets, but as giving them something more than Medicare: a personal financial stake in their use of necessary healthcare. But there is also a public interest argument to recommend demand-side focused health reform.

The real priority for states is to save themselves from the financial and political calamity of Medicare by securing genuine reforms that address the health system's financial integrity. State governments could save themselves from Medicare's problems by taking back their tax powers and reclaiming their authority over public hospital policy. States need to acknowledge how they can become champions of genuine structural change in the public health sector. Health system affordability relies on the demand-side intervention; so in the interests of fiscal and political self-preservation, states should recognise the gain from becoming advocates not only for rational federalism, but also for pairing such interventions with a cost-sharing (and potentially a 'health savings') approach to health financing. To save themselves from Medicare and to make public hospitals affordable, states ultimately must encourage their citizens to contribute to the cost of their own health care.

It is frequently observed in relation to the health debate that Australia needs an honest and open national conversation about the future of its health system to address unrealistic community expectations about the constraints that dog a 'free' health system. Most governments and politicians, federal and state alike, avoid this subject; they live in fear of the electoral consequences of belling the cat about the true limitations of Medicare. Yet at the state level especially, by the time rampant public hospital demand eventually culminates in uncontrollable hospital budgetary overruns in the face of intractable waiting times, dissembling will no longer suffice.

Sustainable provision of hospital services would be possible under a rational federal system of devolved income tax and health responsibilities, which include reform on the demand-side that embrace cost sharing—if not within the shield of a 'health savings' vehicle, then at least within a stand-alone, compensated environment. Either option would preserve horizontal equity and enhance the financial integrity of hospital services without jeopardising universality of coverage.

But to create an affordable health system, the collective cultural expectations that surround a 'free' healthcare must yield to the principle of greater personal responsibility for health. This is diametrically opposed to the expectation that normally prevails in public life in Australia: that governments must do all things for all people. Because this expectation can never be fulfilled, it nourishes deep-seated popular distrust of the political process.

The popular perception, therefore, is that politicians are cynical partisans, susceptible to raising false expectations in pursuing their self-interested agendas. The political class in general repays public disdain by treating the average voter as a complaining mendicant with an insatiable appetite for government entitlements. The mutual disregard and contempt between politicians and voters is consecrated by unfulfillable slogans such as 'free hospital care for all'. Looking ahead, the continued operation of 'free' public hospital systems in Australia will almost certainly require a combination of higher taxes, higher deficits and debt, and greater rationing—with cuts to health and other services. As the 'credibility gap' between the promise of 'free' health and the reality grows, it will magnify and potentiate voter disenchantment with politicians.

The chasm between perception of private gain and public good is always vulnerable to exploitation by populism. This creates fertile territory for public disaffection with government. Populists protest loudly (often on single issues) to harvest the discontent of disillusioned voters, but are bereft of solutions. However, political opportunists could prosper by filling the void left by 'establishment politicians' afraid to admit Medicare has defects that require remedies which may be electorally distasteful. Saying and doing nothing about Medicare will leave the governing parties in Australia vulnerable to populist assault over health while ever the demand and cost pressures seem destined to remain uncontrollable. The political class can either allow themselves and their successors to remain hostages to fortune—or to exercise the foresight to pursue owning both the problem and solution to the future of the public hospital system.

To avoid the former fate, politicians must cease gulling voters with the unattainable and acknowledge that 'free' hospital care can never occur. Australia is unworthy of a political class that habitually beguiles voters with falsehoods about the panacea of Medicare, and doggedly panders to them as inherently selfish and venal. If such base expectations come to lie at the heart of the democratic process, it will surely govern how politicians and voters behave towards each other. Health reform presents an opportunity to reassert a civil society in which government becomes truly responsible to the people, and consents to share the burdens of real self-government by, of, and for the people.

The only recourse open to state governments to save themselves from the financial blight of Medicare is by advocating rational federalism and genuine reform in health, and entering into 'hard conversation' with their electorates about the future of public hospitals. To make public hospital systems sustainable, state government must urge citizens to accept greater personal responsibility for health through co-payments and implement cost-sharing strategies. The real reform challenge is to enlist the help of the people to realise this goal. Instead of encouraging voters to ask what public hospitals can do for them for 'free', politicians need to start asking citizens what they can—and must—do for public hospitals.

Endnotes

1   Reform of Federation White Paper – Discussion Paper 2015 (Canberra: 2015), 9-10.

2   Reform of Federation White Paper, 11.

3   http://www.aph.gov.au/About_Parliament/Parliamentary_Departments/Parliamentary_Library/pubs/rp/BudgetReview201617/Hospital

4   'States adopt Morrison's private health model', Sydney Morning Herald, 25 November 2015.

5   John Daley and Cassie McGannon, Budget pressures on Australian governments, 2014 edition, Grattan Institute.

6   Australian Institute of Health and Welfare, Health Expenditure Australia 2014-15, Table A10 70

7   Australian Institute of Health and Welfare, Hospital Resources 2014 -15, Table 4.4 48

8   Australian Institute of Health and Welfare, Elective Surgery Waiting Times 2014-15, Table 2.6 12

9   http://www.smh.com.au/nsw/mike-bairds-four-year-gst-consensus-plan-20160131-gmhyqf.html

10 Productivity Commission, Efficiency in Health, Research Paper, (Canberra: 2015), 31-2.

11 Reform of the Federation White Paper, p.1-6

12 Sidney Sax, A Strife of Interests: Politics and Policies in Australian Health Services (Sydney: George Allen & Unwin, 1984), 73–75.

13 T.H. Kewley, Social Security in Australia, 1900–72 (Sydney: Sydney University Press, 1973), 358.

14 Anne Crichton, Slowly Taking Control?, as above, 134–135.

15 Jeremy Sammut, How! Not How Much: Medicare Spending and Health Resource Allocation in Australia, Policy Monograph 114 (Sydney: The Centre for Independent Studies, 2011).

16 Sammut, How not How much

17 Access Economics, Comparative Effort in Health Financing by the Commonwealth and State Governments (Canberra: 1998).

18 Jeremy Sammut, Why Public Hospitals are Overcrowded: Ten Points for Policy Makers, Policy Monograph 90, (Sydney: The Centre for Independent Studies, 2009).

19 Stephen J. Duckett, "Hospital payment arrangements to encourage efficiency: the case for Victoria, Australia", Health Policy (1995), 34:2:113-134 http://www.sciencedirect.com/science/article/pii/016885109594014Y

20 John Daley, Budget Pressures on Australian Governments (Melbourne: Grattan Institute, 2013).

21 John Graham, The Past is the Future for Public Hospitals: An Insider's Perspective on Hospital
    Administration, CIS Policy Monograph 102 Papers in Health and Ageing (9) (Sydney: The Centre for Independent Studies, 2009).

22 David Gadiel and Jeremy Sammut, 'Health,' in David Clune and Rodney Smith (eds), From Carr to Keneally: Labor in office in NSW 1995–2011 (Allen and Unwin, 2012).

23 NSW Inter-Generational Report 2016, (Sydney: 2016), 10, 80.

24 "Health budget storm as spending to surge past $25bn", The Australian, 13 December, 2016.

25 'Mike Baird makes new case for 15% GST', Sydney Moring Herald, 1 February, 2016.

26 2015 Intergenerational Report Australia in 2055, (Canberra: Commonwealth of Australia, 2015).,

27 Jeremy Sammut, 'Federalism at a Tangent: Public Hospital Reform', in Sovereignty, Blame Games, and Tony Abbott's New Federalism, CIS Policy Forum 27 (Sydney: 2014).

28 National Commission of Audit, (Canberra: 2014), 149.

29 http://www.smh.com.au/federal-politics/political-news/states-could-collect-income-tax-under-radical-plan-to-be-discussed-at-coag-20160329-gntoar.html

30 https://www.coag.gov.au/sites/default/files/agreements/Heads_of_Agreement_between_the_Commonwealth_and_the_States_on_Public_Hospital_Funding-1April2016.pdf

31 Budget Paper No.2 2016-17, 177. http://www.budget.gov.au/2016-17/content/bp2/download/BP2_consolidated.pdf

32 David Gadiel and Jeremy Sammut, How the NSW Coalition Should Govern Health: Strategies for Microeconomic Reform, Policy Monograph 128 (Sydney: The Centre for Independent Studies, 2012)

33 NSW Health, Fees Procedures Manual for Public Health Organisations http://www.health.nsw.gov.au/policies/manuals/Pages/fees-manual.aspx

34 David Gadiel and Jeremy Sammut, 'Public hospitals aren't free: so charge an accommodation fee', Sydney Morning Herald, 10 June, 2014.

35 http://droit-finances.commentcamarche.net/faq/52499-forfait-hospitalier-2017-montant-et-exonerations

36 Jeremy Sammut, 'Health- Opt-Out of Medicare and Opt-In for Personal Health Savings Accounts' in James Allan (ed.), Making Australia Right: Where To From Here? , (Connor Court: Brisbane, 2017).

37 Gadiel and Sammut, Lessons from Singapore: Opt-Out Health Savings Accounts for Australia, Policy Monograph 140, (Sydney: The Centre for Independent Studies, 2014)

38 Gadiel and Sammut, Lessons from Singapore.

39 Gadiel and Sammut, Lessons from Singapore, 13.

Chapter 8

Opt-Out Health Saving Accounts[*]

David Gadiel & Jeremy Sammut

Health iconoclasm in the United Kingdom and Australia

> As technology advances and people live longer, there is
> no way the healthcare systems of developed nations can
> survive at a reasonable cost with a minimum level of equity
> in provision, without putting individual responsibility and
> public health policy at the centre of the debate.
>
> — Tony Blair[1]

The opening ceremony of the 2012 London Olympics paid unusual homage to a national institution: film director Danny Boyle's tribute to the National Health Service (NHS) famously featured 300 illuminated beds emblazoning 'NHS' across the field of the Olympic stadium. Established by the Attlee Labour government after World War II, the NHS has long been viewed by its advocates as a pinnacle of the British welfare state: no matter what else might be said of their country, since 1948 the people of the United Kingdom have accessed 'free and universal' health care paid by tax.

In recent times, however, the celebrated institution thought to have set Britain apart (particularly from the United States) has been subject to greater scrutiny. The core features of the NHS include no or low levels of 'cost sharing' with patients, and low overall levels of private expenditure

---

* First published as Lessons from Singapore: Opt-Out Health Savings Accounts for Australia, Policy Monograph 128, (Sydney: The Centre for Independent Studies, 2014).

on health care. The absence of user charges for most services, which shifts the money cost of health away from individuals and directly on to public expenditure, is not sustainable. For example, a 2014 report on the future of the NHS by the respected independent health think tank, The King's Fund, not only acknowledged the demographic and other financial pressures on the overstretched UK budget, but also risked sacrilege, boldly declaring that "the whole of current direct expenditure on health and social care, both public and private, cannot be met through public spending." The scale of the financial challenge facing the NHS led the King's Fund report to consider a number of possible responses, including new or extended NHS charges that might apply to those able to meet them. Examples of proposed cost-sharing measures are a £10 charge for GP, practice nurses, outpatient, or accident and emergency visits, and a daily accommodation charge of between £10 and £50 for hospital inpatient treatment.[2]

The UK debate about personal responsibility for health care came as Australia's own 'free' taxpayer-funded health system, Medicare, faces structural, cost and ageing challenges analogous to those confronting the NHS. This in turn has invited national debate about similar initiatives that could require Australians to contribute more to meet the cost of publicly funded health care directly and lessen the increasing burden that health is placing on government budgets.

The debate about the introduction of now-abandoned GP co-payments has inspired considerable political heat because Australia's Medicare, like Britain's NHS, has a special national status. Since 1984, Medicare has sought to guarantee all Australians access to health care mostly without user charges. In keeping with the intention of its founders, Medicare has striven to offer access to a 'universal,' single class of a high quality care for well-to-do and poor Australians alike.[3]

The stated rationale for Medicare was that 'universalism' would avoid a 'two-class' health system that gave the poor access to services of inferior quality. A uniform health system would hence reflect the national ethos of a 'fair go' for all. In reality, the evolution of a 'mixed,' public-private health system, together with the structural flaws that have marred Medicare's design since inception, has failed this egalitarian promise. In practice, Medicare has delivered an ever-increasing cost to taxpayers, rather than its promise of 'free and universal' health care for all.

Medicare: Structure, cost and ageing

Medicare provides on-demand access to non-hospital based medical services without user charges if the provider agrees to 'bulk bill' patients and accepts the Medicare Benefits Schedule (MBS) rebate paid by the federal government as payment in full. With around 85% of GP services currently bulk billed, and approximately 75% of all MBS services bulk billed, 'free' medical care is standard, and individuals contributing to the cost of medical care by paying out-of-pocket charges is the exception in Australia. Medicare also entitles Australians to inpatient and outpatient treatment from public hospitals without charge *at point of access*. The cost of 'free' public hospital care is limited, and the overall cost of the Medicare system contained, by rationing and queuing for public elective surgery. For this reason, Australia's public hospital system, managed by states and territories, is shadowed by a private system as well as by private-paying beds in public hospitals. Private treatment both in public and private hospitals duplicates many types of treatment also delivered from 'free' public hospital beds, and some 47% of the population are willing to hold private health insurance mainly to hedge the risk of public waiting lists.

It is not surprising that Australia's complicated public-private health system encourages costly and inefficient allocations of health labour and capital. The federal government contributes to each of the systems. Aside from its activity payments (which started in July 2014) and fixed contributions to state and territory budgets for public hospital operating budgets, the government also contributes to teaching costs and makes discretionary grants to public hospitals for some capital items; and in an attempt to level the playing field, it also indirectly supports private hospitals by subsidising private health insurance premiums via the private health insurance rebate.

Equally unsurprising are the constant cost and demand stresses in the public components of Australia's health services, driven in part by Medicare's free entitlements to medical services, and exacerbated on the supply side by rigid industrial practices in the public hospital system and the lack of competition in the market for hospital services.[4] Demand and supply factors have contributed to a rapid increase in government spending on public hospitals and significant growth in unrestricted medical benefits paid through the MBS. The federal government has been the fastest growing source of public health expenditure in the past decade, including rapidly increasing spending on the premium rebate for private health insurance.[5]

Currently, more than a quarter of Australian government spending is directed to health care, age pensions, and aged care. Without action to limit spending growth, public spending in these areas is projected to increase significantly over the coming decades, driven mainly by the rising cost of health.[6] The Treasury's *Intergenerational Reports* have repeatedly warned about the sustainability of the various components of Medicare, in conjunction with an ageing population and the associated demands that retention of Medicare in its present form will place on government to increase health expenditure.

Demographic challenges are also at work. Australia's population is ageing. This increases the dependency ratio as the proportion of the working-age population diminishes. Without an increase in Australia's overall productivity, other things remaining equal, the rising dependency ratio due to the ageing population will contribute to a reduced tax base and hence cause an increasing structural deficit. The implication if government health programs are to be maintained and greater rationing avoided without incurring increases in the public debt, is that taxation will have to rise to support increased public spending. Alternatively, if increases in taxation and rationing are both to be avoided, a realistic plan for reform of government spending on health and a redesign of Medicare that is sustainable will be the single most important determinant of maintaining quality health services in the future.

Conventional health policy wisdom
and the Singaporean experience

Debate is polarised in Australia about the future direction of health policy and options for cost sharing. Some proponents of the status quo argue that growth of health spending is no reason for concern: As Australia's aggregate income grows, inevitably we can expect to spend a greater share on services such as health, education and travel—and proportionately less on staples such as food and clothing. As demand for health services for the country as a whole is income elastic (so the argument goes), it thus meets the classic economic definition of a 'luxury good'—even though it may be a 'necessity' for individuals.[7] With absolute growth in the economy, we should therefore be quite capable of accommodating Medicare and its expected call on greater public spending over time through higher taxation.[8] This argument downplays the significance of spending ever-higher proportions of GDP on health by ignoring the opportunity costs of inefficiency in the health sector, and by overlooking political and economic limits to government revenue and spending on health amid competing policy priorities.[9]

Nevertheless, opponents of shifting demand for health services away from government subsidies argue this would simply switch a given demand for funding from Medicare to inequitable private sources, including private insurance. The experience of the United States, where combined public and private spending on health is approaching a fifth of the national income, is interpreted as evidence of the failure and inefficiency of private insurance because of its alleged adverse impact on health costs.[10] Others argue that cost sharing is a tax on sickness[11] and would jeopardise the integrity of Medicare—it would disproportionately affect the poor and chronically ill by inhibiting them from seeking access to primary care. This would then inhibit prevention or the interception of disease or both, and could ultimately have the perverse effect of increasing the workload of the public hospital system, causing the overall health budget to increase.[12]

A comparison between Singapore—the one developed nation with a sophisticated cost-sharing health system—and other developed nations such as Australia, with public and private health insurance systems, fails to lend weight to the claim of an inexorable relationship between affluence and health expenditure. On purchasing-power parity criteria at least, Singapore enjoys a real income exceeding Australia, yet the ratio of health to GDP expenditure in Singapore (at 4.9%) is considerably below Australia's (10%) (Figure 9). This indicates that consumers in Singapore necessarily devote a lower share of their income to health expenditure than those in Australia—either directly out-of-pocket or indirectly through taxation or private health insurance. The difference in health expenditure patterns between Singapore and Australia and other comparable countries is explained by differences in their respective health funding architectures, including the high levels of 'first-dollar' individual accountability in Singapore that distinguishes its health funding from other high income countries.

The challenges of sustainability facing health systems around the world contrast with the low spending on health in Singapore, and have made Singapore and its distinctive health funding and service provision arrangements an object of international attention. Compared with other nations, including Australia, Singapore's health system has delivered comparable First World standards of care and health outcomes at much lower cost—an achievement chiefly attributable to the greater personal responsibility for health expenditures and superior incentives for efficiency that are integral features of the Singaporean model.[13]

Conventional health policy wisdom, drawn mainly from the American experience, is that low public health spending and high private health spending is associated with higher health costs and lower health outcomes. Singapore's experience (Figure 10) shows that low public spending, low third-party (private insurance) spending, and high out-of-pocket spending is cost effective and has not adversely affected health outcomes (Figure 11).

Figure 9: Comparative health expenditure as a percentage of GDP, 2014-16

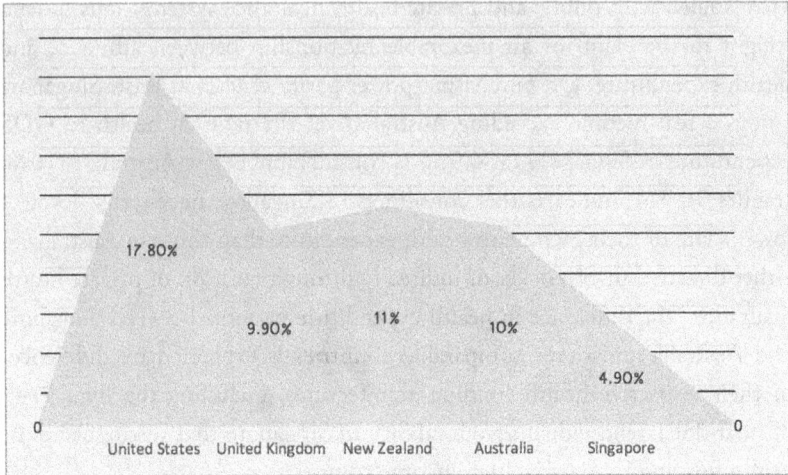

Sources: Centre for Disease Control 2016 (US); Office of National Statistics 2014 (UK); Commonwealth Fund 2015 (New Zealand); AIHW 2015 (Australia); World Bank 2014 (Singapore).

Figure 10: Comparative sources of health expenditure as percentages of total health expenditure, 2014-16

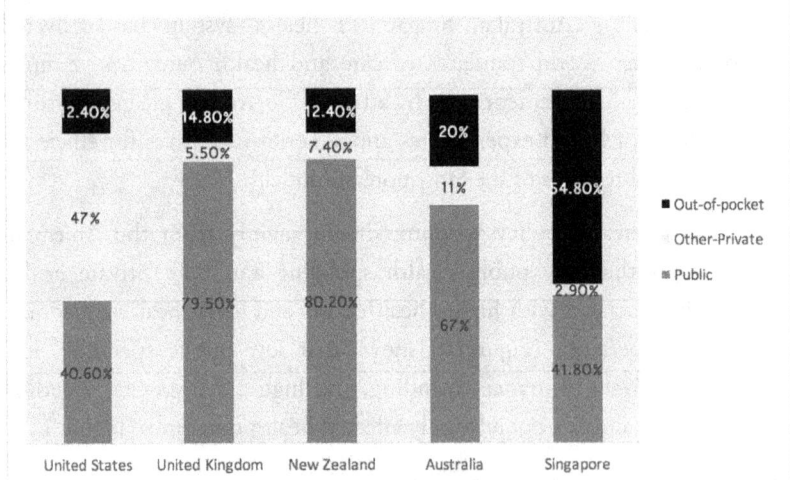

Sources: Centre for Disease Control 2016 (US); Office of National Statistics 2014 (UK); World Bank 2014 & OECD 2016 (New Zealand); OECD 2015 (Australia); World Bank & Trading Economics 2014 (Singapore).

Figure 11: Comparative life expectancy at birth, 2015

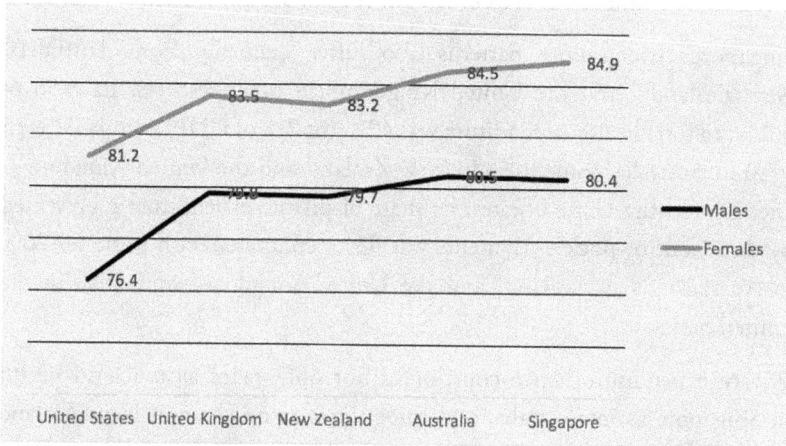

Sources: World Bank 2015.

Comparative health expenditure in Singapore, Australia and other countries

Health system architecture and design influence the services they deliver as well as outcomes that ensue. Studies of comparative health system performance using cross-sectional data are an established field of inquiry.[14] This chapter analyses cross-sectional data on some key health and other indicators in Singapore, Australia, New Zealand, the United Kingdom, and the United States. This invites inter-country comparisons between selected measures of health expenditure, behaviour and outcome.[15]

Although each of the countries selected is comparably affluent with similar health goals, the non-Asian countries mostly organise, deliver and finance their health services in ways that differ markedly from Singapore. In Australia, New Zealand and the United Kingdom, for example, the ratio of total health spending to GDP is typically in the range of 9–11%; in the United States it is 18%. This reflects that apart from the United States, annual per person health expenditure of these countries is AU$7000 – 11, 000. It is at least double that in the United States. Singapore is a rank outlier: it spends 4.9% of its GDP on health and its expenditure per person on

health is less than half that of Australia and slightly more than a third for
New Zealand and the United Kingdom (Figure 12).

Singapore's expenditure patterns also differ markedly from Australia's,
New Zealand's, and the United Kingdom's in other respects. Its ratio of
public to total health expenditure was 42% (or 2% of GDP) compared with
67% in Australia, some 80% in New Zealand and the United Kingdom—
and 40% in the United States; its share of private expenditure represented
by direct out-of-pocket payments was 95%, compared with some 60-70%
in Australia, New Zealand, and the United Kingdom—and 20% in the
United States.

Private expenditure hence contributes not only twice as much to health
in Singapore as in Australia, and three times as much as in New Zealand
and the United Kingdom, but almost all of Singapore's private expenditure
consists of direct out-of-pocket expenditures. Although private expenditure
in Singapore is roughly comparable with that of the United States, some
80% of the latter is covered by third-party payers (private health insurance
carriers).

Figure 12: Comparative health expenditure, selected countries, 2014-15

	United States	United Kingdom	New Zealand	Australia	Singapore
Health expenditure, % GDP (2015)	17.1	9.1	11	10	4.9
Health expenditure per person, AUD (2014)	9403	3935	4896	6031	2752
Per person GDP, Purchasing Power Parity (PPP), international dollars (2016)	57,467	42,609	39,059	46,790	86,856
Public Expenditure % total health expenditure (2014)	48.3	83.1	82.4	67	41.74
Out-of-pocket expenditure % of private expenditure (2014)	21.37	53.1	62.6	57.1	94.1

Sources: All data from World Bank 2014 and World Health Organisation 2015 except for Australian health
expenditure from AIHW 2015.   *Expenditure in US currency extrapolated from AUD data using the
average currency conversion rate of 2013-14 fiscal year.

Why Singapore's health costs are lower than Australia's

Parallels and contrasts

Singapore and Australia share many aspects of their British heritage. Nearly half the population in Singapore speak English at home. It is the only Asian country joined to the Anglosphere.[16] The legal and parliamentary systems of Singapore and Australia share common traditions, and there are recognisable parallels between aspects of their health systems. Undergraduate medical training in the two countries is similar, and before Singapore developed its own system of postgraduate medical education through its School of Postgraduate Medical Studies in 1969, Australian colleges had played an important role in developing Singapore's specialist training program.

Like Australia, Singapore has public and private hospitals and its hospitals attract significant public money. Public hospitals also play a dominant role in the health systems of both countries. Singapore's Ministry of Health manages a public system of acute and specialist hospitals across six different clusters; its private hospitals operate independently. The finance of Singapore's health services embodies a variety of redistributive features, although they are different in principle and practice from Australia's Medicare. Where possible, public hospital remuneration in each country is activity-based and Singapore even uses Australian casemix grouping criteria.

Nevertheless as far as the culture, modes of finance, and the operation and management of health services are concerned, there are striking differences between Australia's Medicare and Singapore's so-called '3M' system. Australia's Medicare is wholly tax financed and 'universal,' and is quite remote from anything to do with the compulsory savings arrangements that set Singapore apart.

Figure 13: The 3M system of health finance in Singapore – source, purpose and application of funding

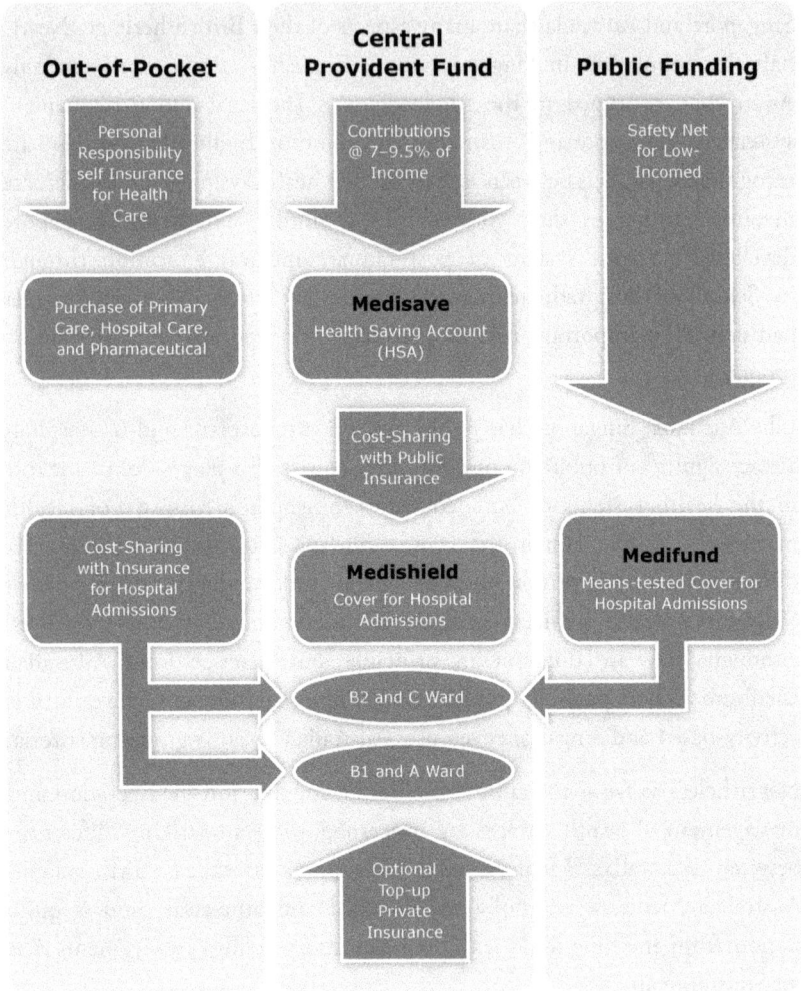

The 3M system

The 3M system—**Medisave, Medishield and Medifund**—is an element in Singapore's method of compulsory household savings that includes health and superannuation, which is administered through its Central Provident Fund (CPF)—a legacy of the British colonial administration. The 3M system is integral to the social objectives of the CPF, and facilitates health goals in harmony with the CPF's mission to help meet population needs for retirement, housing and asset enhancement in a self-reliant manner and without overdependence on taxpayer-funded government support.

Established in the 1980s, the explicit rationale for the 3M system (as set out in the 1983 National Health Care Plan and elaborated in the 1993 'Affordable Health Care' white paper) was to avoid demand and cost spirals that plague other health insurance systems around the world. The aim was to specifically design a system that required people to pay their own way for health so as to control spending on health and keep health care affordable and cost-effective by preventing the overuse that third-party insurance arrangements encourage. Mandating self-reliance was also intended to avoid the rise of an 'entitlement mentality'—the perception of a 'right' to unlimited state-funded care—which is fostered by universal health systems such as Australia's Medicare and Britain's NHS.[17]

The 3M terminology denotes a three-tier hierarchy of household health finance that blends the aims of equity and personal responsibility (Figure 13). Its central pillar is **Medisave**, which is a system of compulsory, age-based income contributions to tax-effective health savings accounts (HSAs), administered by the CPF. Funds accumulated in Medisave HSAs can be used for some specialist treatment and chronic care and for the cost of inpatient hospital care; they may also be used to purchase high-deductible hospital insurance (or to purchase additional private hospital cover) through **Medishield**, the state-run health insurance fund. The third tier, **Medifund**, represents the safety net of the 3M system. It is a government endowment fund providing means-tested payment of the hospital costs of low-income citizens.

Medisave

Medisave payments, in conjunction with government subsidies to public hospitals and polyclinics, are the core element of Singapore's health finance. Most working people in Singapore contribute (with their employer's assistance) between 7% and 9.5% of their salary (depending on their age) to their individual Medisave accounts. Self-employed people are individually assessed for their contributions. Apart from personal and employer contributions, government contributions can also be made to Medisave accounts through the standing grant it pays into the accounts of all newborns—analogous to Australia's erstwhile Baby Bonus.

Medisave represents the health component of a suite of contributory ledgers that the CPF maintains for every Singapore citizen or permanent resident. They remain portable across jobs and into retirement. Besides Medisave, the other CPF saving accounts are a Special Account for retirement-related financial products and an Ordinary Account for purchasing a home or to pay for education. At the age of 55, the balances of savings in an individual's Special, Ordinary and Medisave accounts are rolled into a Retirement Account, subject to a minimum residual threshold remaining in the Medisave account (SG$49,800 in 2016). Retirement Account balances are then used to purchase a lifetime annuity from CPF Life.

CPF contributions are tax exempt, as are withdrawals and income accruing. Although prices in Singapore have remained relatively stable, CPF money is not inflation-proof. Investors receive a bond rate pegged to the prime rates of the largest local banks, returning a guaranteed minimum 4% interest and an additional 1% for combined Medisave, Special, and Retirement Account balances up to SG$60,000. At death, CPF funds, including Medisave balances, can be paid in cash to nominated beneficiaries, free of estate duty.

Limits apply to the total amount that persons may hold in their Medisave accounts (SG$52,000 in 2017). This removes any incentive for account holders to overspend on health. Amounts exceeding the limit automatically flow to Special Accounts (for persons under 55) or to Retirement Accounts.

In 2016, there were some 3.4 million Medisave accounts with a total balance of SG$82.1 billion.[18]

Medisave allows for a risk-control strategy within families. Shortfalls in a Medisave account may be replenished with payments from cash out-of-pocket or by accessing funds in the Medisave accounts of a spouse, parent, child or grandchild. Older patients make frequent use of their children's accounts. Such transfers are believed to be in the spirit of filial piety and 'Asian values.'

Medishield

'Family risk pooling' contributes to the efficiency of the system; it is not a substitute, however, for general risk pooling available from insurance—or national risk pooling as might occur under a properly funded national scheme such as South Korea's,[19] but this is not really a feature of Medicare in Australia (see below). Funds in Medisave accounts may nevertheless be safeguarded from catastrophic risk by using them to pay a premium to purchase Medishield. This is a basic public hospital insurance policy underwritten by the CPF. The Medishield table is subject to deductibles and co-insurance that can be met directly from Medisave balances or out-of-pocket cash. Use of Medisave funds to purchase first-dollar health insurance is prohibited.

Holders of Medishield usually enhance their basic cover by also purchasing an Integrated Shield Plan, which is offered by five approved private medical insurance scheme (PMIS) carriers. Held in conjunction with Medishield (but administered by a private carrier), a higher plan augments Medishield benefits (analogous to private cover in Australia) by paying for superior public wards or for inpatient and other treatment in private hospitals. Integrated Shield/PMIS plans nevertheless also remain subject to deductibles and co-insurance. Even in the most subsidised wards, the patient must pay at least a fifth of the cost.

Some 75% of Singaporeans hold Medishield cover in conjunction with Integrated Shield/PMIS plans. Certain private insurers write non-PMIS insurance plans, but these remain outside the scope of Medishield, and are generally individual or group medical plans specifically offered to expatriate employees. Since 2008, this form of cover became mandatory for all foreign workers, coinciding with the removal of subsidies for foreign workers in public hospitals and polyclinics.

Medisave money is automatically applied after the age of 40 until the age of 65 to the purchase of an Eldershield disability insurance plan. Just over 1 million Eldershield plans provide cover for monthly cash benefits for up to a maximum of 72 months (depending on the level of cover) in the event of disablement. Eldershield Supplements are available for those seeking higher levels of disability cover.

Medifund

In Singapore, there is entirely separate provision for identifying and targeting need and for assisting the indigent to access public health services. Unlike Australia, Singapore has never aspired to universalism through a one-class health system for everybody. Although Singapore has committed to a 'floor' in health care by way of its Medifund, its objective is equity rather than equality.[20]

Medifund is constituted as a government endowment scheme. Subject to means-testing and medical social worker authorisation, it provides charity-style relief for the hospital costs of vulnerable people experiencing hardship. It is supplemented by Eldercare and the Community Health Care Assist Scheme (CHAS). The former subsidises voluntary organisations in delivering services to needy seniors; the latter offers means-tested subsidies to Singapore citizens for GP and dental visits.

Paying for health services in Singapore

The key to Singapore's capacity to restrain health costs is the way the 3M system blends public funding for health services with sources of private savings that are quarantined for the purposes and needs of health and retirement, combined with heavy reliance on out-of-pocket payment for most medical services.

Singapore has restrictions on which health services may be funded from Medisave accounts, and service-specific limits apply to amounts that can be drawn down. Funds may be expended directly on hospital inpatient care (up to SG$450 per day or other prescribed limits for various types of surgery) as well as on day surgery, some costly outpatient treatments, and—at the primary care level—on immunisation and specified chronic disease management. With their own savings at stake, households are encouraged to make judicious choices about health services they use.

To control costs, Singapore tends to be a late adopter of new high-cost technologies. In the case of the supply of public hospital services, there is also direct rationing through government control over public hospital spending. Singapore's private hospitals are not bound by the public system's regulatory environment, although they compete with public hospitals as well as with each other.

However, supply of out-of-hospital GP, specialist and allied health services is mostly free of government intervention. Rationing is left to the price system because most of Singapore's medical care outside hospitals, unlike in Australia, is supplied in a free market, paid for directly out-of-pocket, and accessed primarily in a market-driven GP system, supplemented by competing government-operated polyclinics.

Medisave is designed to encourage a discipline of saving for unforeseen or high-cost health events. It is not intended to provide financial relief from high-frequency, low-severity contingencies amenable to self-medication or to primary care management by a GP or by an allied health professional or the like: these services must be incurred as out-of-pocket expenses. Similar restrictions apply to most prescription pharmaceuticals, which are paid for directly out-of-pocket (minus a government subsidy for listed medications). Although the Singapore government subsidises the price of pharmaceuticals on its list, there is no counterpart to the significant entitlements and safety net arrangements available on Australia's PBS.

The principle of patient financial responsibility is extended to the use of all inpatient hospital treatments in Singapore, where cost must either be met wholly from direct cash out-of-pocket, or Medisave money, or alternatively cost shared on Medishield or on a higher table by way of co-insurance and a deductible. There are special circumstances in which in the case of inpatient care or for ambulatory medical care from a polyclinic, first-dollar coverage may apply for the indigent through Medifund or through CHAS.

Demand side factors in Singapore: Avoiding moral hazard

Although most econometric research indicates that health consumers are responsive to price, evidence of the effect of price on various health market aggregates (such as doctors' visits, length of hospital stay, and hospital separations) is not overwhelming.[21] Demand is nevertheless likely to be more sensitive to the relatively high levels of across-the-board cost sharing evident in Singapore.

The aggregate evidence in Figures 9, 11, and 12 indicates that Singapore's health pricing at the point of consumption may have encouraged consumers to make considered health choices by weighing, at the margin, perceptions of the worth of incremental care against the value of alternative consumption preferences. This has likely caused consumers in Singapore to become extremely familiar with symptoms amenable to self-care, distinguish conditions that are minor or self-limiting, and discriminate effectively between services that are discretionary and those absolutely necessary (and for which it follows that demand is price inelastic).

By contrast under Medicare's 'universalism' in Australia, consumers are largely shielded from direct exposure to the true cost of most health services. Indiscriminate public first-dollar coverage introduces an element of moral hazard, whereby the existence of insurance (in whichever form) may cause some people to use health services for which they would have been unwilling to pay, had they not possessed an insurance entitlement. Singapore's minister of health once famously remarked how Australia's health insurance system (among others) is 'fraught with over-consumption and over-servicing.' He described it as the 'the buffet syndrome of abuses'[22]—a remark that has now entered the lexicon in Singapore as a metaphor for the perils of first-dollar coverage on health services and its association with the risk of moral hazard.[23]

Where demand is price inelastic (as, for example, in the case of insulin for diabetes), moral hazard risks diminish, since demand for care is governed solely by the probability of falling ill. Singapore's policy of targeting full coverage for essential services — such as for immunisation at the primary care level — hence contributes to welfare and efficiency gains.[24]

Without cost sharing, where demand is at all price elastic, moral hazard will likely cause the costs of insurance for most people to exceed the cost of self-insuring for the risk of a health event. This can augment demand, resulting in an overproduction of health services and a deadweight loss to the economy. It becomes one of the main arguments for scrutinising the Medicare philosophy of guaranteed free public entitlement. Indiscriminate entitlements are likely to be associated with inefficiency, inflated health expenditures, loss of welfare, and an even higher demand for insurance.[25]

Inflated health expenditures will be occasioned not only by the increased volume of services demanded but also from bidding up provider fees and wage and salary costs. The implicit publicly funded premium hence embodies double components: premium for genuine risk cover protection and premium to pay for the extra resource cost of moral hazard—even though there may be individual welfare gains from decreased risk bearing.

Supply side factors in Singapore: Incentives for efficiency

Risks of health service overproduction are amplified at zero prices where there is excess supply-side capacity. Government in Singapore hence reinforces the effect of pricing on health service demand by rationing public hospital capacity—the source of 80% of Singapore's hospital bed days. Figure 14 reveals that Singapore's acute bed endowment of 2.1 per 1,000 persons was considerably below Australia's 3.8 and leaner than other countries. In conjunction with cost sharing, rationing reinforces a low claims experience for insurers: Singapore's hospital separation rate of 0.08 per person per year (in 2012) and its hospital drawing rate of 0.51 bed days compares with Australia's respective separation and drawing rates of 0.41 and 2.36.[26] Australia's hospital drawing rates, conditioned by styles of medical practice and supported by first-dollar public and private third party payers, remain among the highest in the world.

Competition policy in Singapore has also helped the 3M system thrive, both as it applies to the operation of public hospitals as well as a consequence of scrutiny by the Competition Commission of Singapore into doctor fee setting practices.

Keeping the costs of health services low and price competitive has made Medisave-funded health care affordable as well as contributing to the overall efficiency of the Singapore health system. In relation to public hospitals, although Singapore's Ministry of Health monitors expenditure on capital items as well as the introduction of new technologies, each public facility operates with more autonomy than tightly and bureaucratically controlled public hospitals in Australia.[27] Although publicly subsidised, Singapore's 16 public hospitals operate as separate corporate entities across six different clusters, with a right to accumulate surpluses and savings, provided they are retained for the benefit of their patient catchments. Their boards are completely independent and not tied into the rigid industrial practices of public institutions to be found in Australia.[28]

This means Singapore builds and operates hospitals cost effectively; its hospitals can respond flexibly to changes in consumer demand (subject to overarching government policies); and the management and organisational structures of its hospitals enable them to deliver services efficiently (across a geography that is admittedly limited compared with countries such as Australia) at lower cost than in Australia. This accounts for the government's overall low share of total health expenditure remaining at some 42%.

There is also price competition for health services in Singapore. Since its foundation as a free port, Singapore has long established a culture of enterprise and price signals.[29] The Ministry of Health nurtures hospital price competition by maintaining a website that publishes information on the range of bill sizes that consumers may expect to incur in public hospitals for different treatments and interventions.[30]

Since May 2004, the ministry has encouraged hospitals to advertise their fees and services. Individual public hospitals maintain their own websites on which they publish their fees for different classes of ward accommodation and other services such as ICU, day theatre fees, and outpatient attendances.[31] There are significant variations in prices charged. This may be attributable to scale of operation, varying management practices, location or market power accruing from professional reputation, and client perceptions of quality and performance.

Public hospitals are always likely to play a dominant role in Singapore, even though they coexist with a vigorous private hospital industry. In Singapore, it nevertheless remains government policy to encourage a contestable private system that can challenge public sector provision. This is evidenced by the structure of non-hospital care that is paid for, out-of-pocket under Medisave.

With regard to medical services, about 80% of Singapore's primary medical care is by private GPs or private medical chains, independently setting their own fees in a private market. The remainder is from 18 publicly operated and subsidised polyclinics—used mainly for chronic conditions, dental care, and immunisation. Cost sharing on consultations and prescriptions nevertheless still applies. Even though fees may be lower than for private GPs, waiting time for an appointment may be longer.

Specialist care is from specialist outpatient clinics in both public hospitals and private hospitals (without needing a GP referral).[32] As in the case of other out-of-hospital care, the cost of all non-inpatient specialist care (including an unsubsidised patient component of public specialist treatment) must be met from direct cash out-of-pocket rather than Medisave balances.

Unlike Australia, direct cash payments by patients are the exclusive source of GP income in Singapore. Doctors cannot set fees with reference to a task-specific benefit payment, which under Medicare in Australia, is taken for granted as a benchmark for fee setting. Neither is there scope for Singapore doctors to recommend fees through their professional associations, as occurs through the Australian Medical Association (AMA) and professional societies in Australia. In 2007, (as Chapter 6 explained) the Singapore Medical Association (SMA) withdrew its *Guideline of Fees* (in force since 1987) to avoid the risk of contravening Singapore's *Competition Act*. In 2010, in recognition of the harm that fee recommendations can do to competition, the Competition Commission of Singapore subsequently affirmed the SMA's action.[33]

Because most of it is paid for out-of-pocket, the market for medical care in Singapore is more competitive than Australia's. Pricing not only plays a role in encouraging health consumers to make discriminating choices, it also constitutes an incentive for practitioners to keep their costs down and to maintain affordable charging practices within the means of a clientele paying for services out-of-pocket.

Primary care practices compete for custom on price, waiting time (most GP private clinics are walk-ins), patient satisfaction, and convenience. Health consumers in Singapore will tend to shop around until they find a practitioner they feel offers good value for money. All GP clinics and many specialist practices also stock medicines and compete as 'one-stop shops' with pharmacies and polyclinics.

The market for primary medical care in New Zealand bears some resemblance to Singapore's. No recommended fee is available in New Zealand and co-insurance applies. In Christchurch, a typical GP visit costs around AU\$30–40 in 2013 and more for out-of-hours, usually AU\$60. A typical Canterbury GP receives roughly half its income from patient contributions.[34]

Like medical care, prescription medicines in Singapore must be paid for directly in cash out-of-pocket—although the government pays a subsidy on a formulary of listed drugs. Some practices compete on consultation price by using their prescription dispensing businesses to cross-subsidise their other work, to the extent that some even believe doctors have become medicine sellers with a licence to prescribe.[35] The notion of a 'two-sided' market for pharmaceuticals and medical services would be quite alien to Australia, accustomed as it is to a strict division of labour between dispensing and prescribing.[36]

Figure 14: Comparative health usage, selected countries, 2012-16

	United States	United Kingdom	New Zealand	Australia	Singapore
Acute hospital beds per 1,000 population	2.8	2.7	2.8	3.8	2.1
Acute separations per person	0.13*	0.27	0.15*	0.41	0.08*
Acute hospital bed days per person	0.7#	0.57	0.3#	2.36	0.51
Doctor visits per person	4.1	5	3.7	7.6	1.7

Sources: OECD 2014 and 2016; US International Trade 2016; Ministry of Health (Singapore) 2012; CDC (US) 2014; Commonwealth Fund 2016. *Data (2010) for all diagnostic categories, not necessarily strictly 'acute'. Manually adjusted from per 100 k persons to per person from stats.oecd.org/ [Health>Health Care Utilization>Hospital aggregates].

HSAs and health status

A test of Singapore's health funding efficiency relative to Australia would be to assess the veracity of the assertion that cost-sharing discourages access to care and thereby causes deterioration in health status.

The Rand Health Insurance Experiment (RHIE) addressed this question in the United States by conducting a random economic experiment over the period 1974–82 to assess the effect of various health insurance policies on the demand for health services and health status.[37] Households were randomly assigned to different cost-sharing groups. To control for adverse selection, each was paid a lump sum to ensure the experiment did not make them worse off. The experiment not only found that people of all ages who contributed more to the cost of their health bills purchased less health services, but also that measured on a variety of criteria, there was no statistically significant measurable difference in health status associated with their higher consumption of services.[38] Yet households that were fully insured consumed 40% more care than those who paid directly for their care.

The experience of the Rand experiment, together with the cross-sectional data comparing the extent of Singapore's cost sharing and broad indicators of health status with those of Australia and other countries, suggests that the design of health insurance is of great consequence to the efficient use of health services. Although Singapore's population admittedly is still comparatively young (only 12% of the population is older than 65 years), the relative scores for vital health statistics identified in Figure 15 indicate that Singapore is generally a healthy society. Its life expectancy at birth is superior to Australia's and that of other comparators, and its infant and under-5 mortality rates are substantially below those of other countries. While Singapore's life expectancy at 65 is lower than Australia's, it is equivalent or superior to those of other countries.

Singapore's low cost health funding and efficient delivery structures, along with the associated high standard of its health outcomes, appear to be serving its clients well. In 2000, in an exercise it has been wary to repeat, the WHO produced a ranking of its 191 member countries on a series of critical scores for public health that included outcomes, responsiveness, fairness of financial contribution, and health expenditure per head. Singapore was placed at 6 and Australia at 32. The United States was close a call at 37 and the United Kingdom scored 18.

Advocates of Singapore's health funding model are legion, despite the limited examples of success with HAS funding models in other countries.[39] (See Box 15) Nevertheless, various writers have alluded to Singapore's Medisave or a variant as a possible role model for Australia to consider—or at least to distil from its broad funding architecture a design for principles of cost sharing and supply-side competition that could be applied to Medicare or to an alternative to Medicare.[40] This could, as a starting point, in turn invite a review of the wisdom of some of the taxpayer-funded universal entitlements available to all Australians justified by either the principle of targeting public support or liberating consumers by enabling greater choice of health cover.

Despite failing to deliver on its equalitarian promises, Medicare remains a 'sacred cow' of iconic proportions, quarantined from reform mainly due to a matrix of vested interests that underpins the politics of health.[†] A bolder and broader approach to funding health reform in Australia that drew heavily on Singapore's experience with HSAs and greater cost sharing could unshackle health from the politics of populism and fanciful expectations about the durability of Medicare. If such change were successfully insinuated alongside Medicare without compromising its 'path dependency'[41] or needlessly alienating its essential constituency, it could become a growing point for compelling more radical systemic change.

Figure 15: Comparative health outcomes, selected countries, 2016

	United States	United Kingdom	New Zealand	Australia	Singapore
Life expectancy at birth, M/F	76.4/81.2	79.8/83.5	79.7/83.3	80.5/84.5	80.4/84.9
Life expectancy at 65, M/F	18/20.6	18.8/21.3	19.1/21.4	19.4/22.2	19.0/22.4
Infant mortality per 1,000 live births	5.6	3.9	4.7	3.2	2.1
Under 5 mortality per 1,000 live births	6.5	4.2	5.7	3.8	2.7
Pop > 65 years, %	15.03	18.35	15	15.25	12.40

Sources: World Bank 2014, 2015 & 2016; OECD (Australia) 2014; Ministry of Health (Singapore) 2016.

† Medicare's protected status rests largely on its capacity to unite a wide spectrum of stakeholders—even though they may possess apparently contradictory goals: by shielding doctors averse to business risk from exposure to the free market, it underwrites private, fee-for-service income; its over-prescriptive Schedule of Services on which medical benefits are paid is costly to maintain, thwarts technological change, and inhibits labour substitution; its guaranteed hospital and medical entitlements can protect uncertain health consumers even from the most trivial and minor health events; it offers employees in public health systems secure careers, insulating their generous award conditions and outdated work practices from market forces; and it represents a source of great pride to advocates of social justice who regard all forms of cost sharing as taxing ill health or encroachments upon entitlements that should be universal. For government, all that remains is funding responsibility.

Box 15: HSAs in other nations

- The health system in Singapore is unique in the sense that its 3M HSA model has been uniformly adopted as its national system. The United States, South Africa and China have introduced HSAs as partial, optional platforms within a variety of broader health funding arrangements. As in Singapore, these HSAs have been constituted as pre-tax 'savings for health' vehicles, coupled with high-deductible tables. In no other jurisdiction, however, have HSAs developed into the dominant force in funding health, comprehensively integrated with retirement savings, as has occurred in Singapore.

- HSAs were introduced in 2003 in the United States, and remain a popular tax effective option covering some 30 million people, but their destiny may be thrown into obscurity as the *Affordable Health Care Act* ('Obamacare') gradually takes effect. This legislation mandates minimum payout ratios and maximum deductibles to an extent that could ultimately compromise the competitiveness of HSA plans and adversely affect their marketability.

- In South Africa, there is no legislation that dictates a design for health insurance. This has led to the evolution of an assortment of HSA innovations with varying levels of deductibles as well as bonuses for participation in preventive health activities. Of the 20% of South Africans who are affluent enough to purchase private health insurance, roughly half purchase HSA cover. However, HSAs remain a 'boutique' offering in a two-class system where the majority of the population rely on a free, overloaded public system.[42] HSAs in South Africa have become a marker for its dual economy and have little chance of making further headway.

- In 1998, China sought to emulate the success of Singapore by introducing HSAs as a component of the basic health insurance system for urban workers in its 50 largest cities. As the first large urban centre to implement them, the experience of Shanghai seems to indicate that urban China may find it difficult to reproduce Singapore's HSA success.

- The main reasons include Shanghai's older and less prosperous population with a rate of unemployment higher than Singapore's. This has limited the uptake of HSAs because the poor do not earn enough to contribute to HSAs. Furthermore, starved of public subsidies, public hospitals in Shanghai have been obliged to draw down patient savings exhaustively, causing a deteriorating HSA experience. This problem has been aggravated because the Shanghai model excludes family risk pooling so that individual accounts face exposures greater than in Singapore. Finally, the tradition of personal accountability, as practised in Singapore, is alien to China whose citizens have been acculturated to publicly provided social largesse.[43]

- It has not been possible elsewhere to replicate national success with HSAs to the extent in Singapore. Critics argue that Singapore has made them work 'but only as one small part of an extremely complicated system involving extensive government intervention.'[44] From this, it could be argued that it may be unwise for Australia to borrow a model found simply to work in Singapore's unique social and city-state geographical setting. It is nevertheless evident that there are particular or local systemic reasons that explain any doubts and uncertainty about HSAs in other countries. This is not a general argument against them.

Agenda for health and superannuation reform in Australia

The existence of a price at the point of consumption in Singapore instils levels of personal responsibility for health that are unknown in the Australian health system. With their own money at stake, Singapore's citizens are encouraged to make judicious choices about using health services. This has contained the cost and increased the affordability of health care, while increasing the overall efficiency of the Singapore health system. With their own money at stake, Singaporeans devote less than half the amount of its GDP to health than Australia, and 60% of health spending is private expenditure. Importantly, this achievement has not detracted from health outcomes and quality of care as Singapore's life expectancy and child mortality data demonstrates.

Australia could draw upon Singapore's Medisave and Medishield as an alternative method of health funding by linking tax effective HSAs, where possible, with the existing superannuation system. At the moment, Australia's occupational superannuation is bound by a set of rigid rules that generally preclude a beneficiary from accessing any benefits until after retirement or transition to retirement. After retirement, opportunities for contributing to superannuation are limited, but since a beneficiary drawing a pension may just as well apply their accumulated savings to health or health insurance as to any other area of their choice, *de facto*, their entitlement can function after retirement much in the same way as a tax-efficient HSA.

It is in the pre-retirement, inflexible and user-unfriendly accumulation phase that scope for building up a separate accessible provision for current health service use offers an ideal opportunity to give health consumers with account-based superannuation plans, so-called 'taxed' funds, a greater stake in funding their own health care.[45]

Like Singapore, Australia has a compulsory contributory private superannuation system, as well as a parallel tax-financed government pension system for those with insufficient savings—but at that point, similarities between Australia and Singapore end. Singapore's superannuation is a government monopoly, defined contribution scheme operated by the CPF that covers the entire workforce. In Australia, superannuation is a mixture of generally unfunded government schemes for public servants and lower income earners; privately operated trusts of various types that may compete with each other for custom; and self-managed funds which are trusts that may include up to four beneficiaries.

Funded, account-based schemes in Australia, mostly privately operated, maintain a ledger on each beneficiary, as in Singapore, but they are discrete from Medicare's unfunded, pooled liability for paying the cost of claims for health service use by the general population. The integration and flexibility of arrangements for retirement saving and health in Singapore are different from the rigid dichotomy that exists in Australia between contributory occupational superannuation for retirement and funding for health services. This is notwithstanding that for retirees on private pensions who hold private health insurance, the distinction between the sources of expenditure becomes increasingly blurred, as retirees in Australia are at liberty to apply their savings to fund increasing use of all manner of services, including for their health.

Funded account-based superannuation schemes, which are highly tax effective savings vehicles, could provide a stepping stone to health funding reform analogous to the Singapore model. Their narrow remit, however, would need to be expanded beyond the current 'sole purpose test.' This restricts their role to providing benefits to their members upon their retirement, and specifically precludes a member deriving a direct or indirect benefit beforehand even if, with large account balances, they may be confronted during their working lives with serious financial problems arising from ill health or temporary disablement.

For young members of the workforce whose retirement could be many years distant, access to their savings to meet current health expenses would motivate them to take a greater interest in their superannuation, and become less lethargic and more discriminating about choosing their fund, if its purposes became less restrictive and amenable to their more immediate needs. The Australian superannuation industry, on the other hand, appears preoccupied with maximising the volume of funds under its control and quite unsympathetic to the principle of early withdrawal, even where households are adequately provisioned.[46]

Medicare opt-out HSAs

A new vision for funding health care in Australia based on the Singapore model could be achieved by applying the principle of choice for those who wish for an alternative to Australia's taxpayer-funded universal health care system. This model could involve some modification to the sole purpose test in conjunction with an increase in the contributions to superannuation during a member's working life. This could fund a medical/hospital accumulation reserve, constituted as a separate but linked HSA, within each member's superannuation account. Members would be able to draw upon these funds during their working lives to meet the cost of specified health expenses in much the same way as under Medisave in Singapore. Upon retirement the medical/hospital accumulation reserve would merge with the pension fund, as occurs in Singapore. The aggregated accumulations would then function exactly the same way as superannuation does now in the pension phase—and, to the extent they were adequately funded, could be applied to self-insurance or alternatively to purchase private health insurance.

This model would offer an alternative to Medicare. It would require individuals to choose to opt into an HSA and trade their Medicare entitlements in exchange for the right to access their tax-efficient medical/hospital accumulation reserve. Figure 16 provides a summary of how a possible opting out arrangement might work. The opting out principle has been canvassed by CIS Senior Fellow, Peter Saunders.[47] Saunders distinguishes between 'entitlement' opt outs and 'contribution' opt outs. He argues that the former embodies a redistributive factor; the latter would simply return people their own money, leaving the poor no worse off. In exchange for their Medicare entitlement, those opting out would have their Medicare contribution (the levy and a component of their income tax) credited to the funding of an annual Health Voucher equivalent to total average per person government spending on health, indexed—approximately $4,600 in 2014-15[‡]—for deposit in their HSA (see Figure 16).

Health Voucher money that was unspent would accumulate from year-to-year and the interest accruing might attract the same 15% concessional tax rate as income in taxed superannuation funds for retirement during their accumulation phase.

In the United States, HSA holders are relieved of all income tax, so there may be precedents for treating health balances more generously than retirement balances.

HSAs could be maintained during the accumulation phase of a superannuation account and kept separate from, but linked to, the pension component during a beneficiary's working life.

Part of the trade of Medicare entitlements for HSAs would be that in exchange for control of one's own health dollars, individuals would agree to save up and take responsibility for their own health care costs in retirement. Health vouchers would cease when pension eligibility age is reached. This means HSAs would yield long-term savings to government by establishing non-government sources of funding for old age health costs.

---

‡ In 2014-15, average per person health expenditure in Australia was $6,846,. This includes money spent on health services by individuals from their own pockets and money spent paying for services insured privately or funded through Medicare. The government-funded share of total health spending was 66.9% or $4,579.97 per person. AIHW (Australian Institute of Health and Welfare), Health Expenditure Australia 2014–15 (Canberra: AIHW, 2016), 31, Table 2.6.

The mechanics of debiting a health bill to an HSA would be similar to lodging a claim with Medicare or a private health fund. Health funds are accustomed to processing large volumes of frequent transactions associated with conventional indemnity claims. They would be well equipped to maintain and remit expenses debited to HSA balances to service providers— either as providers in their own right or as contractors to superannuation funds. Pooled HSA reserves accruing from unspent Health Voucher money would function like earmarked personal bank accounts. They could be managed by approved organisations such as registered health funds or superannuation funds. Their balances would merge with retirement savings once a pension commenced.

The embodiment of the financial incentive from assuming personal responsibility for health services, currently received and paid for by tax at zero prices at the point of consumption, would accrue from the financial benefit of cashing out Medicare entitlements and using cost-effective HSAs, funded by Health Vouchers. As well as the tax concessions, the benefit would include savings from lower premiums for high-deductible insurance that eliminated the inflated costs of first-dollar cover and moral hazard— all of which would eventually accrue to individuals in the form of higher superannuation balances and retirement incomes. A potential indirect effect of HSAs, therefore, could help limit future calls on the public pension.

Since the value of Health Vouchers would remain fixed regardless of any tax contribution to Medicare, they would offer equity between different classes of taxpayers. This would avoid the objection often levelled at HSAs in the United States that they provide disproportionate gains to persons wealthy enough to benefit from the tax concessions and offer nothing to those who pay no tax. The advantages accruing to Australian HSA holders would thus not be limited to those paying tax: the incentives accruing from Health Vouchers would be available to welfare and high-income earners alike, even though, because of the redistributive factor, they might each attach a different value to the potential gain.

HSAs would introduce a new tax-effective regime of private provision and accountability for health not possible under current Medicare arrangements, since individuals claiming against their HSAs would become personally liable for their own health care expenses. Since Medicare entitlements were being cashed out in return for assuming personal responsibility for health, there would be no restriction on the use of HSA funds to pay for approved primary care, and specified prescription pharmaceuticals, as in Singapore. Those joining HSAs will in fact have traded their Medicare benefit entitlement for their Health Voucher.

High-deductible insurance tables, available in conjunction with HSA models, such as Singapore's Medishield, would offer the benefit of risk pooling for an account holder's exposure to outlier high-cost claims involving hospital or day surgery or specified high cost pharmaceuticals, prostheses and appliances, and the cost of managing chronic conditions. By eliminating the overuse problem associated with first-dollar health insurance, HSAs keep health cover affordable by reducing the premiums charged for high-deductible health plans. It is likely that a new market for similar type tables for catastrophic and chronic conditions would develop in Australia, probably offered through existing registered health insurers or other institutions operating HSAs on behalf of their holders.

HSA holders accordingly could choose to apply part of their balances to pay premiums for HSA high-deductible private health insurance if they wished. Their contributions could vary according to the standard of cover and level of entitlement purchased, which could be subject to varying limits and exclusions. All HSA health insurance policies would need to be non-cancellable, and carriers should not have the right to refuse to accept an application for cover. Front-end costs of deductibles, including approved GP services, would be met from HSA balances or, if they were insufficient or could not be met from a close relative's account balance, paid with out-of-pocket cash. HSA carriers would seek to negotiate new service contracts and preferred provider arrangements for their members covered for treatment in both private hospitals and public hospitals.

Figure 16: New vision for health funding in Australia

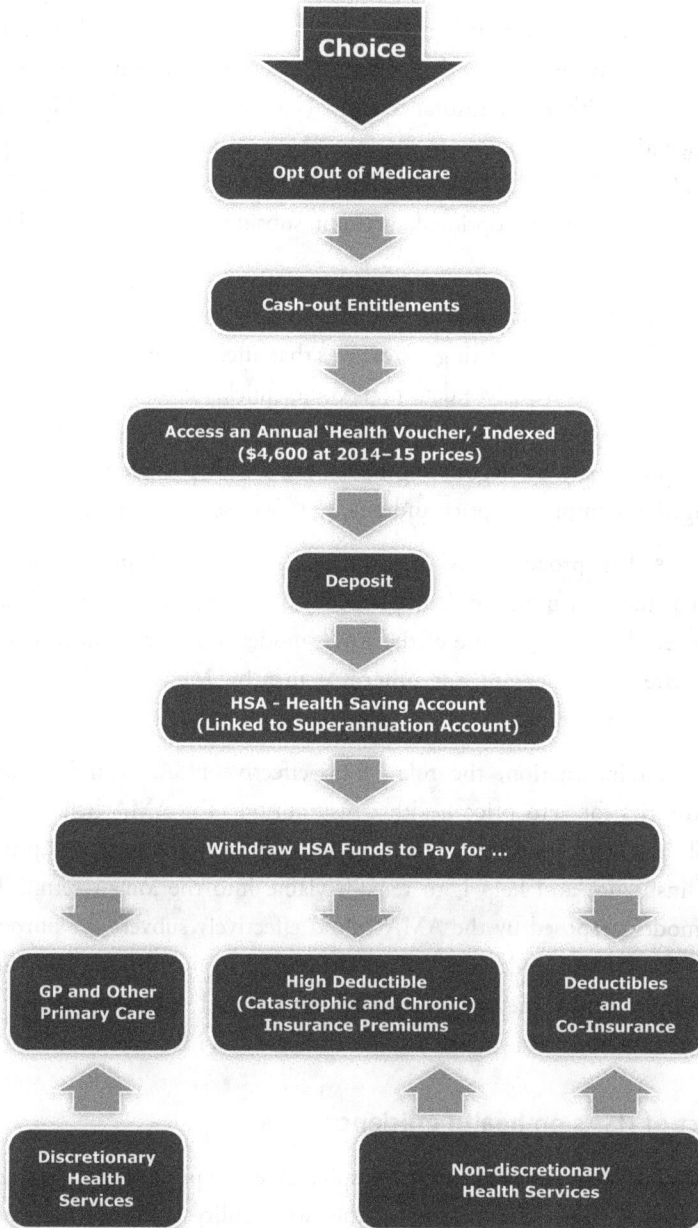

Choice

Opt Out of Medicare

Cash-out Entitlements

Access an Annual 'Health Voucher,' Indexed
($4,600 at 2014–15 prices)

Deposit

HSA - Health Saving Account
(Linked to Superannuation Account)

Withdraw HSA Funds to Pay for ...

| GP and Other Primary Care | High Deductible (Catastrophic and Chronic) Insurance Premiums | Deductibles and Co-Insurance |

Discretionary Health Services

Non-discretionary Health Services

Upon first entry into the opt-out scheme, a transitional arrangement will be needed to protect a small minority of individuals experiencing exceptional health events from exhausting their HSA balances before they could accumulate. This should take the form of a subsidised government-operated catastrophic health event insurance fund (such as for specified high cost pharmaceuticals) with low cost sharing. The premium would be charged to the Health Voucher for a compulsory initial three- to five-year period. Thereafter, it would be optional, without subsidy, and subject to higher cost sharing.

It may take time for the impact of HSAs to flow through the health care market and remove the existing distortions that affect prices, but all insurers could be expected to analyse data that would quickly enable them to move into the high-deductible market to offer better value for money for HSA holders, principally by negotiating better deals with providers who would be obliged to compete on price and quality to win service contracts.

The AMA has proposed its own version of a contributory HSA for Australia that purports to 'complement' Medicare and private health insurance. The main purpose of the AMA model is 'to meet out-of-pocket health care costs that are not otherwise met by Medicare, the PBS or private health insurance.'[48]

In such an incarnation, the role of tax-effective HSAs would enhance opportunities for zero price health consumption. The AMA believes that 'a well-designed system of HSAs could strongly complement private health insurance and help it to remain viable into the longer term.' The HSA model proposed by the AMA would effectively subvert the purposes for which HSAs were designed. By contributing to moral hazard, it could serve only to inflate the cost of medical services and ultimately contribute to the destabilisation of private health insurance and Medicare.[49]

Impact of HSAs on health efficiency

Supply-side competition for out-of-hospital care and prescription medicines in Singapore has contributed to the workability and acceptance of

Medisave. In turn, Medisave shapes the competitive environment as much as it reflects it.

If Australia were to emulate the Singapore model with new cost sharing options for funding health as an optional alternative to Medicare, it would help drive greater supply-side competitiveness. Australian HSA holders would further this process by assuming private liability for most of their front-end primary care, apart perhaps from essential, price inelastic services such as immunisation and specified high-cost pharmaceuticals.

Providers would start to recognise the importance of catering to the needs of an emerging clientele attracted into cost-effective HSAs, and who took a much keener interest in the cost and content of their care. If numbers or concentrations of patients within metropolitan geographical areas were to defect to HSAs, doctors in these catchments could be obliged to compete for custom by practising outside the boundaries of the rigid service descriptions of the MBS. This would have the potential to create local contestable markets involving fee discounts, new competitive and innovative service packages, and other forms of non-price competition.

Nurse practitioner labour could become more freely substitutable for medical labour as competition became a driver for legislative change; midwives would gain more responsibility for obstetric work; allied health would compete more aggressively for the first-call of patients; self-care and preventive forms of lifestyle would become greater priorities; and greater all-round health workforce flexibility would help mitigate doctor 'shortages.'

A non-NHS market for some prescription medicines could germinate. In Singapore, originator brands now account for less than a third of the market in their respective therapeutic classes as against nearly 60% on Australia's PBS.[50] An HSA market would further the acceptance of generics, as cost-conscious HSA subscribers sought value for money.

The monopoly long enjoyed by community pharmacies licensed to dispense PBS medicines under Section 90 of the *National Health Act* would atrophy. Non-NHS pharmacies would become more viable, and notwithstanding the resilience of the pharmacy lobby, this competition could ultimately become a stepping-stone for general retailers to enter the business of retail pharmacy. There may also be a greater call on pharmacist labour, as community pharmacists hone their skills in 'front-of-shop' work in a bid to compete with other primary care providers.

All of such labour market shifts occasioned by a contestable market in HSA primary care could be expected to contribute to greater flexibility and efficiency in the delivery of health services without (as attested by the Singapore experience) necessarily compromising service quality or health outcomes. Cost-sharing and service privatisation would reduce moral hazard and contribute to reducing the generational burden of Medicare. Moreover, as health practitioners started to standardise their service offerings to all classes of their clientele, and because of the interdependence between the labour markets serving competing HSA and Medicare systems, the efficiency effects of HSAs would gradually filter through to the labour and service markets of the health economy serving Medicare itself.

Implications of HSAs for health insurance in Australia

A HSA system would be fundamentally different to a Medicare Select-style scheme, but it would also facilitate insurance and payment reforms along similar general lines. A HSA system would also permit health funds to operate as financial risk holders and integrated care managers, responsible for catering for the chronic and catastrophic care needs of HSA holders by acting as informed purchasers and negotiating service contracts and preferred provider arrangements on behalf of their new, cost-conscious clientele. As an alternative to Medicare Select, HSAs would also avoid the need for the complex risk-rating of health insurance vouchers that are an essential feature of that model. Nor would it require the community rating of insurance premiums, which currently allows insurers to shift the cost of high risk patients on to a secondary re-insurance risk pool.

As part of the equity principle associated with community rating for traditional private health insurance, private health insurers at present are required to share the cost of high risk contributors by participating in a national reinsurance pool, the Reinsurance Trust Fund. This shelters funds with a disproportionate share of bad health risks by attempting to spread risk equally and avoid chronic market instability.

Since HSAs are designed to provide incentives for account holders to modify and improve their health and claiming behaviours, and to reduce moral hazard, it would be self-defeating to require HSA deductible tables to be part of a risk equalisation scheme—the cost of which would in any case flow through to account holders. Since HSAs would have nothing to do with community rating, their object being to reward privately and encourage self-accountability, there would be no point in requiring tables specifically designed for HSA use to be obliged to participate in a public system that blunted incentives by spreading bad health risks rather than pricing them into the market.

Nor would there be justification to provide a 30% government subsidy for high-deductible HSA tables as occurs in conventional private tables funded from post-tax dollars, since premiums of the former would in any case be payable from tax-advantaged HSA funds, thereby reducing the tax churn. By the same token, it would need to be impossible for HSA holders to simultaneously contribute to conventional private tables: Once a health consumer had chosen to opt out of Medicare, they would automatically surrender their right to access any form of first-dollar coverage or a government-subsidised private health insurance table. Any public subsidy to HSA tables would obviously contribute to moral hazard.[51]

No health fund would be allowed to deny cover to HSA-holders based on health status. But rather than community rating, bad risk would instead be priced into the cost of insurance premiums to encourage funds to properly manage the care of their members, contain benefit costs, and keep premiums competitive and affordable. Hence, the likely innovations a HSA system would spur include the efficiency and quality improvements with respect to enhanced chronic care, and the effective management of access to specialist care in hospital and outpatient settings. Hence, HSAs would not only address moral hazard through the use of prices across the entire health system to control demand; they would also be a contestable market for more efficient and cost-effective provision of insured health services—with the efficiency effects on the supply-side enhanced as providers compete on price and quality to satisfy customers spending their own health dollars to access care.

Eliminating the inflated cost of moral hazard and over-insurance would improve overall health system affordability, including by lowering the cost of health insurance premiums. HSAs would also minimise the administrative costs of health insurance by reducing the volume of benefit claims requiring processing, while also reducing the operational costs incurred trying to direct members to preferred provider GPs, specialists and other ambulatory care.

HSAs could also potentially reduce the political obstacles to introducing a greater element of managed care into the portion of health services that would be covered by health funds. HSAs would allow for the retention of self-funded, fee-for-service payments and free choice of doctor for the vast majority of GP and specialist consultations—potentially weakening the medical profession's resolute opposition to the introduction of an element of managed care into the health system. Moreover, GPs could also benefit financially from integrated payment models that rewarded them for managing care efficiently. Allowing GPs to share in the money put back on the table in reducing hospital utilisation would address the disparity between GP and other specialist incomes that has long been a source of tension within the medical profession.

The creation of a genuine private medical practice system — underpinned by patient choice, professional independence, and retention of the 'sacred' doctor-patient relationship — would also help avoid the excesses of early forays into managed care in the United States, where some HMOs sought to contain costs through skimping on care by limiting the range of approved providers and services. These concerns about denial of access and lack of choice of doctor are at the heart of the campaign techniques used by the AMA to foster public concern and political timidity around the subjects of insurance and payment reform. However, HSAs would allow for the appropriate retention of fee-for-service medicine in a real market setting, and for the innovative integration of insured services at the high-cost, high-risk end of the health system—a combination that might smooth the rough political waters that all meaningful health reforms must navigate.

This raises potential objections to HSAs in Australia. Opponents are likely to claim that Singapore-type HSAs would fracture the national risk pool associated with Medicare. According to this view, a compulsory national system of coverage, such as Medicare, creates a national pooling of risk, which because of its diversity and spread, is the most efficient way of providing insurance and protecting against catastrophic events.[52] Permitting households to opt out of this risk pool by crediting their Health Voucher to an HSA (including perhaps those persons with a disposition to reduce their claims through behavioural change) would encourage adverse selection and jeopardise the integrity of the risk pool.

On the other hand, although Medicare may give the appearance of a national insurance scheme, it fails to abide by insurance principles. The medical component of Medicare, for instance, is simply an unfunded, open-ended budget liability—it has no connection with insurance in the true sense of the term. It offers a guaranteed first-dollar hospital benefit entitlement; for out-of-hospital services where doctors bulk bill, it embodies very little in the way of effective loss control or supply-side monitoring. This prevents effective pricing of overall risk. It is thus very easy for persons with Medicare coverage to surrender at zero prices to a third-party agency arrangement wherein doctors' practice styles may exert influence on the volume of services that is at odds with the principle of consumer choice and sovereignty or consumers' needs. The medical component of Medicare as it stands is effectively no more than a pay-as-you-go rebate program.

There is nevertheless a likelihood of HSA tables eroding the risk composition of traditional private tables currently available through registered health funds. Healthy people who cash out their Medicare entitlements would necessarily be leached from the market for traditional private health insurance as they sought to escape the 'overcharging' that community rating imposes on low risk contributors. Since HSA high-deductible tables would be free to adopt experience rating, they would be open to the accusation of 'cream skimming' and contributing to a redistribution of income towards healthy populations. Under the highly regulated environment in which they operate, private health funds would no doubt regard them as a threat to market stability.

The problem of adverse risk selection could be mitigated by eliminating all forms of first-dollar coverage on traditional private insurance, including the practice of paying 100% of the hospital cost of all private patient stays at public hospitals as well as ceasing to offer medical gap insurance on higher hospital tables. Full gap cover for medical costs can never be guaranteed because health funds have no ultimate control over what doctors may charge. This in turn places continuing demands on gap cover ceilings and could ultimately contribute to the risk of an adverse selection 'death spiral.'[53]

Higher private hospital tables in any case have long become repositories for people who plan or expect to encounter significant private hospital expenses. This is the classic problem of asymmetric information associated with moral hazard where the insured knows more about their risk characteristics than the carrier. At the moment, this exacerbates Australia's comparatively high hospital drawing rate; it thereby inflates the cost of private health insurance and contributes to the overall burden of health expenditure by way of the incremental cost of public subsidies to private health insurance—the fastest component of growth in federal government expenditure on health.

An analogous source of possible objection to HSAs would be that they would destabilise Medicare by fracturing its universalism and lead to a two-class system of health care that arbitrarily created unjust advantages for the recipients of Health Vouchers. These are similar to concerns levelled at private health insurance. To the extent that they have been realised, they may have at least alleviated some of the strain on the public hospital system—and contributed by way of public hospital charges for private patients to an additional stream of state revenue. There are clearly well-established market and political resistances to any draconian attempts to inhibit personal autonomy and health choices in a free society.

State-based HSAs

Singapore-type HSAs could also offer a useful vehicle for states adopting rational federalism (see Chapter 7) to adapt, in different scenarios, to their own respective demand-side strategies for pricing hospital care. Accordingly, states that embraced rational federalism might unilaterally permit their residents to establish HSAs for themselves to pair with their hospital co-payments.

In one scenario, the baseline value of vouchers the state would deposit into HSAs would be limited to public hospital funding, set at per-person state expenditure on public hospitals. Voucher baseline payments would be supplemented with the value of the compensatory payment that would automatically apply to everyone in the state to neutralise the impact of default hospital co-payments, regardless of whether they established an HSA.

Voucher funds would be also supplemented with accumulated superannuation-style contributions deposited into the HSA during a person's working life. Households opting out of their states' Hospital Medicare would transfer their public and their private hospital entitlements (depending on the level of private insurance) into their HSA, equivalent to not less than the entitlements of households remaining in Medicare. HSA funds could thus be available to pay for all charges arising from both public and private hospital care, including private insurance premiums.

In this scenario, the baseline value of the voucher would be equivalent to public hospital funding in each participating state. Under the proposed revision of federal tax and health responsibilities, states would be directly and solely responsible for determining such funding from amounts collected as state income tax by the federal government on their behalf.

Whereas the cost of the public patient entitlement to hospital care (equivalent to Hospital Medicare) together with co-payment compensation would be fully incorporated in the value of the annual voucher, the cost of insurance for households choosing private cover as an add-on would be debited to account-held savings without compensation, and paid (as necessary) from account-holder contributions.

In summary, all hospital admissions in states concerned would remain subject to co-payments and other cost-sharing as described in the previous section, paid either from HSA balances, or—in the case of those remaining in the default arrangements under state-financed Hospital Medicare—as out-of-pocket expenses. (Figure 17)

Figure 17: Source and application of hospital funding under Rational Federalism

Type and source of funding / Patient status	Default household payment arrangements	HSA household payment arrangements
	State public hospital funding sourced from state income tax (default state system)	Households opt out of entitlement to state hospital subsidies in exchange for an annual voucher funded from state income tax and paid into an HSA account, supplemented with occupational contributions
PUBLIC	Entitlement to free public hospital care as a public patient, subject to co-payment (compensated), paid out-of-pocket	Entitlement to public care in public hospitals with liability for state subsidised public fees, paid either out-of-pocket, from HSA money or from health insurance (purchased with HSA money) plus co-payment (compensated), paid either from HSA money or out-of-pocket
PRIVATE	Entitlement to private care in public hospitals, with liability for state-subsidised private fees raised by public hospitals paid either out-of-pocket or by private health insurance, plus private insurance co-payments / cost-sharing (compensated at the public rate), paid out-of-pocket	Entitlement to private care in public hospitals with liability for state subsidised private fees paid either out-of-pocket, from HSA money or from private health insurance (purchased with HSA money) plus private insurance co-payments / cost-sharing (compensated at the public rate), paid either from HSA money or out-of-pocket

In another more comprehensive scenario, states could implement HSAs by incorporating all Medicare expenditure into the value of the voucher. This would require both the state and federal governments to cash out their entire Medicare spending for households opting for HSAs into a jointly-funded voucher that could be integrated into the new division of federal-state responsibilities. Federal government agreement to include the federal government's 'own program' Medicare expenditure on the MBS and PBS in the voucher could then be negotiated as components of the state income tax package. The illustrative per-person value of an annual HSA voucher under each of the scenarios is shown in Figure 18.

Figure 18: HSA Vouchers ($) 2014-15

	State + Federal Public Hospital ($ billion)	Per Person State + Federal Public Hospital	Federal Health (MBS & PBS) ($ billion)	Per Person State & Federal Public Hospital + Federal Health
NSW	13.11	$1,697	9.79	$2,965
VIC	10.08	$1,662	7.06	$2,825
QLD	8.13	$1,678	5.72	$2,858
WA	4.82	$1,841	2.53	$2,809
SA	3.55	$2,080	2.08	$3,298
TAS	1.00	$1,936	0.65	$3,204
ACT	0.98	$2,482	0.37	$3,416
NT	0.75	$3,075	0.20	$3,900
Aust.	42.44	$1,759	28.41	$2,937

Source: Australian Institute of Health and Welfare, Health Expenditure Australia 2014-15 Report, Tables B27, B30, B33, B36, B39, B42,B45, and B48 of Appendix B; Table A6 of Appendix A http://www.aihw.gov.au/publication-detail/?id=60129557170&tab=3

There is much to recommend in incorporating HSAs into the Australian health system. Allowing individuals to self-fund their own healthcare and to save over time to pay for health would contribute to off-budget, non-tax sources of health funding, thereby reducing health-related fiscal pressures on government budgets. In Singapore, for example, government health spending accounts for 42% of total health expenditure compared to 67% in Australia.

In addition, households and government would financially gain both from lower resource costs flowing from containing the moral hazard effects of wasteful and excessive service demands, and from supply-side discipline exerted upon public hospital managers. Insofar as such savings accrued to households in the form of higher HSA balances that merged with superannuation balances on retirement (as occurs in Singapore and proposed in the CIS model), they would be available to fund both rising age-related health costs and/or retirement incomes.

There are analogies between the principle of employing superannuation-style account-based savings vehicles as a stepping stone to health funding and the application of voluntary superannuation contributions to assist in purchasing a first home. Tax effective assistance for home purchase through superannuation became available to Australians from 1 July, 2017.[54] Like health savings accounts, the notion of housing assistance accounts is borrowed from the Singapore CPF model of superannuation. For young members of the workforce whose retirement could be many years distant, access to their savings to meet current housing needs, if it were available in conjunction with a similar arrangement for health purposes, would constitute a new savings suite that could further motivate them to take greater interest in their superannuation earlier in their lives and to become more discriminating about their choice of fund to serve their more immediate needs.[§]

A choice-based health reform alternative to Medicare

Singapore's successful experiment with HSAs relies on a complicated and intricate series of mechanisms operating through its CPF, carefully targeted government funding, and a societal consensus. Its health system is unique

---

§ We offer no opinion as to use of superannuation savings as a policy to address "housing affordability". Our argument relates to the general principle of broadening its use as a source of savings other than for the "sole purpose" test as defined in s62 of the Superannuation Industry (Supervision) Act 1993.

in the sense that its 3M HSA model has been uniformly adopted as the national system together with its superannuation.

In conjunction with direct rationing through government monitoring of public hospital spending, and rationing through the price system for out-of-hospital care, Singapore's 3M health finance model of cost sharing has helped it become a world leader in efficient and effective health service delivery. It offers a model that attracts increasing attention from other high-income countries.

The personal disciplines and accountabilities that are a corollary of the 3M system go hand-in-hand with the peculiar combination of a tolerance of government intervention and supply side control in conjunction with autonomous, competing public hospitals and market-driven GP and specialist behaviour.

The destiny of HSAs in other countries that have to date implemented them as partial, optional platforms is uncertain for explicit systemic reasons that do not constitute barriers in Australia. An optional HSA model in which participants cashed out their Medicare entitlements hence remains an opportunity for Australia.

There are parallels between the superannuation mechanisms of Australia and Singapore, except that the Australian occupational system of private superannuation is at present limited to the purposes of retirement and cannot be accessed beforehand. Australia's established pattern of contributory savings could be broadened to accommodate Singapore's cost sharing mechanisms in health in conjunction with a right to opt out of Medicare entitlements.

To the extent that Australia has gone some way towards privatising the public pension system by shifting from Pay-As-You-Go taxpayer funding to Save-As-You-Go self-funding for retirement, there are good reasons on the grounds of sustainability and efficiency to emulate this transition for health services by diluting the monopoly of Medicare.

Medicare opt-out HSAs have the potential over time to establish substantial non-government sources of health funding and take pressure off government budgets by limiting future exposure to rising health expenditure. The effect of exits from the universal system could relieve pressures on the public hospital system as well as on the cost of medical and pharmaceutical benefits; it would also create a drive towards a more competitive health economy in which there were more effective price signals in both labour and service markets. The private health insurance industry could benefit from new lines of business in HSA account management as well as in writing new HSA high-deductible tables, and there would be savings to the federal government's subsidies for private health insurance. Existing registered benefits tables may nevertheless experience some backwash without measures to arrest anti-selection. This could be a spur to their redesign and to a review of all forms of gap cover. A review of the government's mandate of 100% cover for the hospital costs of private patients treated in public hospitals would also be a priority.

An overhaul of the various components of Medicare would be timely. Since its introduction in October 1984 it has remained remarkably intact, apart from a series of fine tunings at the margin that have extended certainty of entitlement (thus adding to moral hazard) by way of safety nets for high claimants and various incentives to encourage GPs to bulk bill. This has entrenched Medicare as a monopolistic service for everyone—rather than targeting need and conserving resources for the poorest and most vulnerable.

While it is unusual for a country to introduce fundamental change to the way it finances its health care, it is important that the design of Australia's health system bears some relation to the demographic challenges it confronts, as well as representing overall value for money. Opt-out HSAs offer a politically feasible path to health reform not only due to the element of choice — since those who do not wish to can stay with Medicare — but also because of who would emerge as the winners from this reform process. Medicare as it stands will be unsustainable without a lift in health productivity, or more taxation, or more public debt, or some combination of these. One obvious alternative to consider is the way in which Singapore has nurtured a low cost, competitive health economy in which HSAs have flourished, and allow Australians to opt out of Medicare and assume personal financial responsibility for self-funding their own health care.

Endnotes

1   Tony Blair, A Journey: My Political Life (London: Arrow Books, 2011), 660.

2   Kate Barker, A New Settlement for Health and Social Care, Interim report of the Commission on the Future of Health and Social Care in England (London: The King's Fund, 2014).

3   Richard Scotton and Christine Macdonald, The Making of Medibank (Kensington: University of New South Wales, 1993).

4   David Gadiel and Jeremy Sammut, How the NSW Coalition Should Govern Health: Strategies for Microeconomic Reform, Policy Monograph 128 (Sydney: The Centre for Independent Studies 2012).

5   John Daly, Budget Pressures on Australian Governments (Melbourne: Grattan Institute, April 2013), 16.

6   National Commission of Audit, Towards Responsible Government (Canberra: Commonwealth of Australia, 2014), 189.

7   Elasticities might be small within Australia, but as it becomes more affluent as a nation, Australia will deliver greater quantities of care with superior technologies. Thus, at a country level, health can be a 'luxury' but a 'necessity' at individual and market levels. T. Getzen, 'Health care is an individual necessity and a national luxury: Applying multilevel decision models to the analysis of health care expenditure,' Journal of Health Economics 19:2 (2000).

8   Ross Gittins, 'The spin behind growing health costs,' The Sydney Morning Herald (29 January 2014).

9   Jeremy Sammut, Saving Medicare But NOT As We Know It (Sydney: The Centre for Independent Studies, 2013).

10 Jennifer Doggett and Ian McAuley, 'A new approach to health funding,' D!ssent 42 (2013). The impact of high levels of insurance coverage is complicated in the United States because of the effects of its malpractice system in stimulating defensive medicine. With insurance, to be sure, neither patients nor physicians bear most 'over treatment' costs, but aside from administrative costs a significant component of the source of the excessive costs of care in the United States resides in its tort liability environment. Daniel Kessler, 'Evaluating the Medical Malpractice System and Options for Reform,' Journal of Economic Perspectives 25:2 (2011).

11 Jeff Richardson, The Effects of Consumer Co-payments in Medical Care, Background Paper No. 5 (Melbourne: National Health Strategy, June 1991).

12 Jennifer Doggett and Ian McAuley, 'A new approach to health funding,' as above; Stephen Duckett, 'Happy birthday, Medicare. Now, how can we make you better?' The Australian Financial Review (31 January 2014); John Dwyer, 'Harsh cuts won't help our health,' The Australian (16 May 2014).

13 A general introduction to Singapore's health system is to be found in William Haseltine, Affordable Excellence: The Singapore Healthcare Story (Washington, DC: Brookings Institution, 2013)—on which material the paragraphs that follow draw, in conjunction with information available from the Ministry of Health Singapore; https://www.moh.gov.sg/content/moh_web/home.html.

14 WHO (World Health Organization), The World Health Report 2000. Health Systems: Improving Performance (Geneva: 2000).

15 Robin Gauld, et. al, 'Advanced Asia's health systems in comparison,' Health Policy 79 (2006).

16 Daniel Hannan, 'Singapore and the Anglosphere,' Speech to the Lew Kuan Yew School of Public Policy, National University of Singapore (3 March 2014).

17 William Haseltine, Affordable Excellence: The Singapore Healthcare Story, as above.

18 Ministry of Health Singapore https://www.moh.gov.sg/content/moh_web/home.html.

19 Soonman Kwon, 'Thirty Years of National Health Insurance in South Korea: Lessons for Achieving Universal Health Care Coverage,' Health Policy and Planning 24:1 (2009).

20 David Reisman, 'Payment for Health in Singapore,' International Journal of Social Economics 33:2 (2006).

21 Jeff Richardson, 'Price Elasticities for Private Medical Care in Australia,' in P.M. Tatchell (ed.), Economics and Health 1982, Proceedings of the Fourth Australian Conference of Health Economists, Health Economics Research Unit, Australian National University (Canberra: 1983).

22 An analogy is where some people overeat at Chinese buffets when the price per meal is fixed. Khaw Boon Wan, 'Fixing our roof,' speech at the Healthcare Cluster National Day Observance Ceremony (17 August 2004).

23 Jeremy Lim, 'Paying for health—the fundamentals are ... fundamental,' SMA News (December 2011).

24 Though even in such limiting situations, counterintuitively, it can be shown that higher levels of utility prevail with cost sharing than without it. Jonathan Baldry, 'Moral Hazard and Optimal Medical Insurance,' in Jonathan Baldry (ed.), Economics and Health: 1998, proceedings of the Twentieth Australian Conference of Health Economists (Kensington: University of NSW 1999).

25 Jeremy Sammut, How! Not How Much: Medicare Spending and Health Resource Allocation in Australia, Policy Monograph 114 (Sydney: The Centre for Independent Studies, 2011).

26 This is a raw, unstandardised comparison that ignores age/sex factors.

27 David Gadiel and Jeremy Sammut, How the NSW Coalition Should Govern Health, as above.

28 Kai Hong Phua, 'Corporatization of Hospitals in Singapore,' in April L. Harding and Alexander S. Preker (eds), Innovations in Health Service Delivery: Corporatization in the Hospital Sector (Baltimore: Johns Hopkins University Press, 2003).

29 David Reisman, 'Payment for Health in Singapore,' as above.

30 www.moh.gov.sg/content/moh_web/home/costs_and_financing/HospitalBillSize.html

31 See, Changi General: www.moh.gov.sg/content/moh_web/home/costs_and_financing/HospitalBillSize.html; Alexandra: www.ah.com.sg/page.aspx?id=138; National University: www.nuh.com.sg/patients-and-visitors/appointments/hospital-charges/inpatient-charges.html

32 The government offers Singaporeans a subsidy of 50% of the cost of specialist care delivered from public hospital outpatient clinics, provided it is referred from a polyclinic or by an accident and emergency department. Specialist treatment at clinics at private hospitals is not subsidised.

33 CCS (Competition Commission of Singapore), Statement of Decision Pursuant to Regulation 9 of the Competition Regulations 2007. Application for Decision by the Singapore Medical Association in Relation to its Guideline on Fees Pursuant to Section 44 of the Competition Act (18 August 2010).

34 Nicolas Timmins and Chris Ham, The Quest for Integrated Health and Social Care. A Case Study in Canterbury, New Zealand (The King's Fund: London 2013).

35 'MOH to stop GP clinics from selling medicine' (Singapore), website.

36 Doctor dispensing is nevertheless a valued source of income in medical practice in many parts of Asia, without evidence, however, of deleterious effects upon health. David Gadiel, Harmacy: The Political Economy of Community Pharmacy in Australia, Papers in Health and Ageing (5), Policy Monograph 89 (Sydney: The Centre for Independent Studies, 2008).

37 Joseph Newhouse, Free For All? Lessons from the RAND Health Insurance Experiment (Cambridge: Harvard University Press, 1993).

38 Cost sharing nevertheless was associated with poorer blood pressure control in low-income groups that though not detected by the experiment, could have been consistent with higher mortality.

39 William Haseltine, Affordable Excellence: The Singapore Healthcare Story, as above; John Spiers, Individual Savings Account Will Improve Access and Performance (London: Institute of Economic Affairs, 2008); Douglas Carswell and Dan Hannan, The Plan: Twelve Months to Renew Britain (London: 2008).

40 David Leyonhjelm, 'Why we should save up to be sick,' The Australian Financial Review (7 February 2014).

41 Gwyn Bevan and Ray Robinson, 'The Interplay Between Economic and Political Logics: Path Dependency in Health Care in England,' Journal of Health Politics, Policy and Law 30:1–2 (2005).

42 Shaun Matisonn, Medical Savings Accounts in South Africa, Policy Report No. 234 (Dallas: National Center for Policy Analysis, 2000).

43 Weizhen Dong, 'Can Health Care Financing Policy Be Emulated? The Singaporean Medical Savings Accounts Model and its Shanghai Replica,' Journal of Public Health 28 (2006).

44 Martin McKee and Reinhard Busse, 'Medical Savings Accounts: Singapore's Non-Solution to Healthcare Costs,' British Medical Journal 347 (2013), 4797.

45 Non-account based schemes (now being phased out) are excluded from this discussion. They are funds that offer defined benefits and are restricted to employees of the provider, mostly in the public sector. Defined benefit schemes that are unfunded and untaxed still exist in the public sector—in contrast to the taxed schemes now offered that are account based, defined contribution schemes.

46 Sophie Elsworth, 'Super raid on our nest eggs,' Sunday Telegraph (4 May 2014).

47 Peter Saunders, The Government Giveth and the Government Taketh Away. Tax Welfare Churning and the Case for Welfare State Opt Outs (Sydney: The Centre for Independent Studies, 2007).

48 file:///C:/Users/setup/Downloads/AMA%20Health%20Savings%20Accounts%20 Policy%20Paper_D09_3402.pdf

49 A parallel proposal to guarantee patients access to out-of-hospital GP services at zero price is being trialled by Medibank Private for persons covered on its hospital tables in SE Queensland at IPN practices owned by Sonic Health (possibly in breach of the Private Health Insurance Act) Sean Parnell, 'Medibank Private to pick up GP costs in trial,' The Australian (10 January 2014). This could have analogous destabilising effects.

50 Hans Löfgren, 'Reshaping Australian Drug Policy: The Dilemmas of Generic Medicines Policy,' Australia and New Zealand Health Policy 4:11 (2007).

51 Petra Steinorth, 'Impact of Health Savings Accounts on Precautionary Savings, Demand for Health Insurance and Prevention Effort,' Journal of Health Economics 30 (2011).

52 David Cutler, and Richard Zechauser, 'The Anatomy of Health Insurance,' in Anthony J. Culyer and Joseph P. Newhouse (eds), Handbook of Health Economics 1 (Amsterdam: Elsevier, 2000).

53 David Cutler, and Richard Zechauser, 'Adverse Selection in Health Insurance,' in Alan M. Garber (ed.), Frontiers in Health Policy Research 1 (Massachusetts: MIT 1998).

54 Budget 2017-18, Fact Sheet 1.4 – First Home Super Saver Scheme. http://www.budget. gov.au/201718/content/glossies/factsheets/html/HA_14.htm

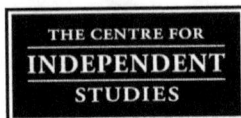

www.ingramcontent.com/pod-product-compliance
Lightning Source LLC
Chambersburg PA
CBHW061140220326
41599CB00025B/4305